PRINCIPLES OF

THE ALEXANDER TECHNIQUE

What it is, how it works, and what it can do for you

2nd Edition

Jeremy Chance

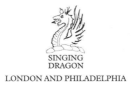

SINGING
DRAGON
LONDON AND PHILADELPHIA

This edition published in 2013
by Singing Dragon
an imprint of Jessica Kingsley Publishers
116 Pentonville Road
London N1 9JB, UK
and
400 Market Street, Suite 400
Philadelphia, PA 19106, USA

www.singingdragon.com

First edition published in 1998 by Thorsons, an imprint of HarperCollins

Library of Congress Cataloging in Publication Data
A CIP catalog record for this book is available from the Library of Congress

British Library Cataloguing in Publication Data
A CIP catalogue record for this book is available from the British Library

ISBN 978 1 84819 128 0
eISBN 978 0 85701 105 3

Printed and bound in Great Britain

Dedicated to my teacher,
Marjorie Barstow
(1899–1996),
and to my dad
(1906–1988)

CONTENTS

Foreword

Jeremy Chance has made a significant contribution to the world of the Alexander Technique with his production and editing for the past 15 years[1] of the high-quality international periodical, *direction*.

Jeremy has also made a significant contribution to the Alexander Technique in Australia as the moving spirit for the establishing of, and as the formulator of the constitution for, the Australian Society of Teachers of the Alexander Technique in 1984.

With this book Jeremy extends his contribution to the Alexander world as a communicator and a thinker in relation to the Alexander Technique.

The book will be of value to teachers of the Alexander Technique as a guide to communicating about the Technique from an expert communicator, as well as providing clear explanations for anatomy and physiology so relevant to the Technique.

To those who know little of the Alexander Technique but who would like to know more, this book is likely to emerge as the most useful exposition of the Technique available. The book is succinct yet comprehensive in setting the Alexander Technique in context, providing the anatomical and physiological basis for the processes of the Technique, describing a lesson (the unique transmission of sensory and motor information between teacher and learner),

---

1 This Foreword was part of the first edition in 1998, and the text has been changed for this new edition. In 2001, Jeremy turned over *direction* journal to be published and edited by Paul Cook. See the Resources section at the end of the book for further information.

the importance of the learner in observing her/himself, as well as an overview of the different traditions in teaching the Technique.

Some leading thinkers and scientists of this century have contributed to the Alexander Technique by their public commendation of the Technique. John Dewey, unstinting in his praise for the Technique, was a seminal philosopher of education and of science in the USA in the early part of the century. Nobel Prize-winning physiologist Sir Charles Sherrington spoke in the 1930s of how impressed he was by the contributions by the layman F. M. Alexander to the understanding of the brain's control of the musculoskeletal system. In the 1970s Nobel Prize-winning ethologist Niko Tinbergen used his prize-winning speech to draw the attention of the scientific and medical world to the importance of Alexander's observations.

This book will make its own distinctive contribution to the Alexander Technique by an expert communicator. I commend the book to all those who wish to know more about a unique Technique which can help restore the sixth sense of proprioception (muscle sense) to the individual and so lead to an improved functioning of mind and body.

David Garlick BSc(Med) MBBS PhD
(1933–2002)[2]

---

2 David Garlick had a long and distinguished career as a medical research scientist, ending as Director of Sports Medicine Programs at the University of New South Wales. Professor Garlick also trained and taught as an Alexander Technique teacher.

ACKNOWLEDGEMENTS

I would like to thank Maureen Chance, William Brenner and Rosemary Chance, my precious and treasured teacher Marjorie Barstow, my students who have helped me develop this information, KAPPA that created the environment to write, Vicki Robinson for her early morning illustrations and Alexander himself.

Extracts from *The Use of Self* by F. M. Alexander, published by Victor Gollancz Ltd, are reproduced with kind permission.

PREFACE TO THE SECOND EDITION

Alexander's discoveries are my passion; they have been my life and work since the age of 20, and I intend to be living and teaching them up to my last breath.

Alexander first started teaching in Australia in the 1890s, yet the impact of his work on modern, mainstream society is hard to fathom or see. Today, Alexander's passionate vision of transforming education and the health of human society has withered away, leaving in its wake a profession that continues on, largely on the fringe; a profession whose members overall are about as much in demand as the actors who wait tables in New York.

A significant number of those who undertake the three years of teacher training[1] will not go on to have a full-time teaching career: they will struggle to find pupils. Some might instead make it their 'hobby'; others think of it as their 'vocation', while keeping their day job; some will co-opt it into their original career as some kind of performing artist. Compared to the numbers who have trained, precious few occupy their lives as full-time professionals. After over 100 years, is this all we can manage? It is deeply disappointing to me.

---

1 Three years is a minimum only; no teacher really understands how to teach the work until they have been practising for many more years. In Japan, the minimum time a person must study before they qualify from our school is four years. The cost is around $40,000 so it is a huge undertaking, and one that I am committed to turning into a viable career.

I believe something is wrong with this picture. If Alexander's discoveries are of such significance – and personally I rank them with the discoveries of Einstein and Newton in terms of their potential impact on humanity – then why do Alexander's discoveries continue to wallow in obscurity? Why does the Alexander Technique mostly manifest in our society today as a non-starter amongst a plethora of modern-day mind and body techniques? Pilates, yoga, acupuncture, hypnotherapy… Most consumers have heard of these, but very rarely have they heard of the Alexander Technique! Why are so many others doing so well, while the work founded by the person that Aldous Huxley described as 'the father of the non-verbal humanities in the Western world' does so poorly?

The answer, I believe, is contained within a nascent 21st-century question that is beginning to pop its inconvenient head into the journals of modern-day science; namely, 'What is human consciousness?' Today there is a coalition of scientific disciplines,[2] collected together under the general denominator of 'cognitive science', which is beginning to challenge the prevailing materialistic view of our world by asking difficult and currently unanswered questions about the true nature of human consciousness.

If the 20th century was all about discovering the nature of matter, then I predict the 21st century will be about discovering the nature of our human consciousness. But this is an altogether different scientific problem, requiring an altogether different methodology to explore it. The idea that knowledge can exist separately from the person possessing it, which lies at the heart of our modern-day research and

---

2   Among these disciplines we can name neuroscientists, philosophers of mind, psychologists, and robotic engineers. Please go to www.alexanderscience.org to find out more on this topic.

education[3] edifice, is finally on the verge of being challenged by mainstream science.

It begins with the emerging discovery by medical science that our mind, in mysterious and unexplained ways, has the power to influence the health of our bodies: through prayer, through meditation, through mere thought alone.

In 1967 the Harvard Medical School began conducting experiments to determine the effects of meditation on our well-being, and has since evolved a theory of a 'relaxation response' as a counterfoil to the 'fight or flight' response we are typically thought to have to stress. The mechanism remains unexplained, but if one follows a certain procedure, the relaxation response can be reproduced every time. To those associated with Alexander's work, this will sound very familiar!

Alexander's work is situated within this emerging coalition of scientists, all working to bring legitimacy to a branch of scientific research dismissed up until now as 'soft and fussy' compared to the 'hard' sciences that explore the material world. The First World War, with its devasation of an entire generation of male youth and destuction of the illusion of an advanced, intelligent civilization, nipped in the bud the blossoming movement led by Western thinkers such as William James and John Dewey and instead ushered in an era of behaviouralism, which only began to be discredited in the mid-1950s.[4] Interestingly, as scientists begin returning

---

3   There is an interesting discussion by Alexander in *MSI* (*Conscious Constructive Control of the Individual*) where he faults the methodology of science for neglecting to include the consciousness of the subject undergoing the experiment. In this way, he anticipated the cognitive scientific assertion, first proposed by Varella, that the state of the person undergoing an experiment significantly affected the result of that experiment.

4   See 'Cognition: A Western Perspective' by Howard E. Gardner, Ph.D. in *MindScience: An East–West Dialogue* by the Dalai Lama, Herbert Benson, Robert A. F. Thurman, Howard E. Gardener, Daniel Goleman and participants in the Harvard Mind Science Symposium, Somerville, MA: Wisdom Publications, 1991.

to these questions, Alexander's name keeps popping up in old literature![5]

Every new scientific advance in our understanding of reality needs an innovation of observation, a new instrument from which to see the world afresh, so that data previously collected but not coherently apprehended can be reinterpreted within a radical new context. Sometimes this new innovation is an object, such as a telescope; sometimes it is a new idea, such as 'the earth is round'.

Alexander's work offers scientists exactly this kind of observational innovation. His simple discovery of a governing relationship between head and spine, which in turn integrates other bodily systems, is so simple it is breathtaking. It explains and organizes data in a way that has not been possible before, offering a previously unknown but now unparalled mechanism for consistently and reliably calibrating the condition of our mental and physical health.

Alexander teachers spend all their time exploring this simple discovery in lessons: how it affects our physical pain and discomfort, our capacity to breathe, our ability to move, our relationships with others, even our ability to think. Alexander lessons practically demonstrate that the origin of this dramatic mechanism – which has such a global, systemic effect on every aspect of our living – lies within the field of our human consciousness; it originates within the way we think. Is thought or consciousness a material thing? If it isn't, what exactly is it? What kind of relationship does this mechanism of consciousness – so demonstratably 'there' – have with the known material world? These are the kind of questions that cognitive scientists are beginning to ask.

---

5   Many of these ideas were first expressed by Rachel Zahn in her appearance at the Seventh International Congress of the F. M. Alexander Technique in Oxford in 2004, summarized in the paper 'Francisco Varela and the Gesture of Awareness' (available at http://alexandertechnique.com/ats/zahn.pdf).

Underlying these questions is a new premise: nothing exists independently from you. Although simple, I am sure you don't think like that. I am sure that you, like me, have been brainwashed into believing that there are things that exist, and can be measured and objectively understood, separately from your own subjective consciousness of that perception. However, practically all materialistic science and research is premised on this assertion of independently existing phenomena.

Or at least that was so until Heisenberg's 'uncertainty principle' hit the scholarly airwaves. He proposed the preposterous idea that the person observing the phenomena affected what was being observed. What happened to 'objective' science, with its idea of independently existing absolutes? From that day, this view of the world started to crumble, and another began slowly emerging to take its place.

The evolving scientific methodology to explore this view, first proposed by Varella, does not go along with the idea that there is separate 'objective knowledge' that can be ascertained independently of the person ascertaining it. Instead, this new methodology assumes that the subject, the experimenter and the objective results – measureable by 'hard science' – are in a relative relationship; therefore, no result of an experimental process can be considered valid unless there is an account of all these factors within that result. If you think about it, that's a pretty radical idea.

And (in case you didn't know it) this is exactly what happens in an Alexander lesson. Your lesson is an experiment in human consciousness, as applied to the problem of the neuromuscular 'coordination' of your system to do 'things'. When I use the words 'coordination' and 'things', I mean them in the widest sense: not just how you move from A to B, but how you problem-solve, how you relate to others, how you handle a crisis, how you breathe. In every instance, 'something' is responsible for coordinating your activity. That 'something' is your human consciousness: a poorly understood phenomenon that sits at the heart of everything we do yet until now has inspired only passing interest within the confines of conventional scientific research. It is an 'eel' of modern science, something that is so ubiquitous it slips away every time we try to look at it. Yet *this* is what Alexander researched; *this* is the subject of your every lesson in the Alexander Technique, and lessons demonstrate conclusively that the cognitive manipulation of this energetic phenomenon can yield immediate and dramatic results.

When you have an Alexander lesson, you can experience significant and amazing new discoveries about the nature of your being. For you, the information will be specific, effective, original and nothing short of revolutionary. Then you leave your lesson and try to explain to your friend what happened. You can't; there are no specific exercises to describe. There is nothing special that you did. It is easy to describe what you do in a yoga class, or a Pilates class, or during your gym training, or while getting a healing of some kind: it is almost impossible to do the same for your Alexander class...

'What did you do in your lesson?'

'Oh, we sat in chair. Then I stood up again. Then we sat again.'

'Oh, really?'

'But it was amazing! I learnt so much.'

'I see.'

If scientific researchers have avoided the question of how to understand and organize human consciousness for so long –

because it is so hard to get a handle on – is it so surprising that mainstream society has difficulty in appreciating the subject? Scientific discovery usually leads the consumer to new things, so if science is lagging, no wonder Alexander's work has proved so unsuccessful in gaining a significant following.

So don't wait too long before you try out what I predict will eventually become the 'next big thing' in the market place of the 21st century.

Tokyo, 2012

1

Introduction

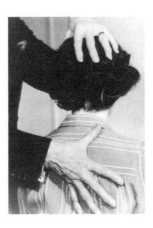

Despite the fact that our posture has significant and long-term effects on our health, we know surprisingly little about how we coordinate ourselves. As you are reading now, how much do you know about your sitting or standing? Do you know how it happens?

I imagine you are sometimes aware of aches or pains? You probably possess a few inherited ideas about what is 'good' and 'bad' about your posture, but I'm guessing nothing very deep or profound. You may know exercises or stretches that help you feel temporarily better, but you keep having to repeat them. Would you like to feel permanently better?

The Alexander Technique is a permanent, on-going solution to the problem of pain brought about by inefficient coordination. If you want to know more about that, you are reading the right book. If you keep reading, it may be that your life will permanently change.

When in real trouble, most of us go to someone for help. Why? Because most of us don't know how to intelligently manage posturally induced pain. So we go to someone who does know: a bone-cracker, a masseur or someone who can do acupuncture or shiatsu. But usually it's rarely permanent – we keep having to go back.

On the other hand, maybe you work out at the gym, or exercise regularly, and feel fit and healthy because of it. What will happen when you get busy, or older, and you stop exercising? Will you stay healthy if you stop?

The Alexander Technique will teach you about a plan for managing your coordination that really works. It is a plan that harnesses your intelligence to bring about an understanding and pleasure in moving that has no equal in the world today.

If you decide to investigate lessons in the Alexander Technique, you are in good company. Some of last century's leading thinkers and icons have studied Alexander's ideas. Starting with George Bernard Shaw, then philosopher John Dewey, writer Aldous Huxley – heard of any of them? How about Sting or Paul McCartney? All have benefited from studying Alexander's discoveries. So did the cinematic Superman, the late Christopher Reeve, who used his Alexander Technique understanding to transform his body from the nervous, agitated Clark Kent, to the magnificent, athletic Superman. It's a nice metaphor for the work: teaching people to become Supermen or Superwomen!

Jokes aside, Alexander's discoveries do teach you a lifelong way of managing your movement that is an education, not a therapy; that puts you in charge of your comfort and ease; that teaches you how to be do things efficiently and well; a technique that offers benefits in areas that seem almost unbelievable, if it weren't for the fact that these changes have been recorded by thousands of people for over a hundred years.

Sounds too good to be true? How about a winner of the Nobel Prize for Medicine – would you believe him?

> From personal experience we can already confirm some of the seemingly fantastic claims made by Alexander and his followers – namely, that many types of underperformance and even ailments, both mental and physical, can be alleviated, sometimes to a surprising degree, by teaching the body musculature to function differently. We already notice, with growing amazement, very striking improvements in such diverse things as high blood pressure, breathing, depth of sleep, overall cheerfulness and mental alertness, resilience against outside pressures, and in such a refined skill as playing a musical instrument. (Tinbergen 1973)[1]

So now I am guessing you are asking the question: what is this all about? And the answer to that question is so simple, it's shocking: we distort Nature's coordination plan, and end up harming ourselves because of it.

This is Nature's coordination plan:

1. Head movements govern vertebral coordination.

2. Vertebral coordination in turn governs the movements of our arms and legs.

But then...

3. We impose our own coordination plan – distorting Nature's plan – leading to unhealthy consequences,

---

1   Professor N. Tinbergen (1907–1988); from his Nobel Oration for the Medicine Prize, 1973.

because our own wrong plan feels like the right plan.

4. Over time our distorted coordination creates a host of physical and mental problems with a variety that boggles the mind.

That's basically the story. We need to get back to Nature's coordination plan. But how? Alexander said:

'You can't tell a person what to do, because the thing you have to do is a sensation.'

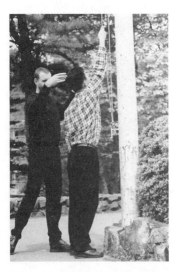

'What you will learn in your Alexander lesson is how you "use" yourself, how you coordinate your body movements to do everyday things.' Photo by Akihiro Tada.

Warning

This book, by itself, is unlikely to transform your way of moving. It will be a support, it will get you thinking, it will make you aware of the problem. I even offer some practical techniques that can bring you insight and benefits. But the problem, the basic problem at the heart of changing our coordination to become reliant again, is our ignorance of our distortion of Nature's plan. We already know Nature's plan – there is no need to learn that. The knowledge is there, hard-wired into us, but it's been imposed upon by so many delusionary ideas about our 'posture' that we have become like the politician who believes his own lies.

We are living a 'coordination' lie, believing it's the truth. Physical troubles originate mentally: our conception governs what happens, not 'our body'. Did you ever hear of a dead body getting a back ache? There has to be a mind there, or nothing happens.

We get so used to splitting our thinking from our body that we talk in lies about ourselves. We say things like 'I have a bad back', but who is making my back bad if not me? 'I make my back bad' is the truth of the matter, but we rarely speak about our physical problems this way. We apportion blame to every possible source (my back, my work, my stress, my partner) without ever stopping to consider that if something is going wrong, then the most likely cause is something *we are already doing* to make it wrong. How can we find out what that is?

The modern world's answer to this question is: *get better by doing more, by imposing more.* This is plainly wrong. We don't find out anything about ourselves by trying to do more; we only confuse things by piling complication upon what is already happening. Instead, like detectives solving a mystery, we must embark on a journey to find *how we are already thinking/moving* that makes our backs in pain or generates general discomfort. As we discover these answers, we simply quit those habits before they give us even more harm. We don't add things; we give up things.

In Alexander's work, we may start out with a 'physical' problem but soon come to see that the problem is *how we think about how we move*. Alexander's discoveries inhabit an in-between world: neither solely about body and physical pain nor solely about mind and psychological pain. Instead, Alexander's work explores the interdependency of these two: how intelligence and reasoning can be applied to bodily coordination. Alexander Technique lessons, through utilizing your intelligence, let you *experience* again the amazing *sensations* of coordinating your body in the way Nature intended it.

Actually, we experienced Nature's plan when we were little, but we forgot that experience. So how do we *re*-experience Nature's coordination plan?

We *re*-experience it through the touch of our Alexander teacher. An AT teacher is trained to touch you in a unique way: they train for over three years so they can know how to use touch to facilitate your *re*-experiencing a *sensation* of movement that is miraculous, because Nature is miraculous. There will be more about this later in the book. The magic of an Alexander lesson comes not just from what you learn but from what you *feel*. No learning is more convincing or quicker than learning that combines intellectual understanding with *kinaesthetic experiences*.

The Alexander Technique, together with its logical side, is *experiential*: it is a *sensation*. And what a sensation it is! You can come out of your lesson feeling like a new person. Your walking is lighter, your head movement freer than you can remember it. You feel as lithe as a cat. And all your Alexander teacher has done, by using his or her hands in a unique and special way, is taught you to restore a coordination plan that was yours to begin with anyway. I doubt you have ever had this happen to you before. I know that because of the look of surprise on the faces of the thousands of people I have helped in my 30 years of teaching.

Want to learn more? Then read on, enjoy your journey into finding out more about who you are and what you are capable of. The best place to start is two centuries ago with the amazing adventures and discoveries of Alexander himself...

2

Alexander's Story

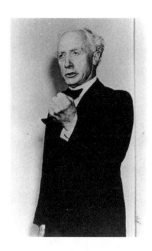

'...my experience may one day be recognized as a signpost directing the explorer to a country hitherto "undiscovered", and one which offers unlimited opportunity for fruitful research to the patient and observant pioneer.'

F. M. Alexander

It all began when friendly actors casually mentioned that they could hear him gasping for air during a performance. Alexander was mortified. Being a bit of a show-off, he prided himself on avoiding this tiresome habit, so common among the 'declamatory thespians' of his Victorian era.

But things got worse. Soon this was the least of his problems, for not only did he gasp for air during his popular performances of Shakespeare's works but on several occasions he lost his voice entirely. In desperation, Alexander sought whatever help he could. Perhaps if it had been London, and not Australia in the 1800s, Alexander may have met a Fogarty – a famous speech coach in London – and today there would be no Alexander Technique. Luckily for us, Alexander was instead within the rough and tumble of a young emerging country and it was every man for himself.

Colonial Australia at that time was imbued with a fighting pioneer spirit which was stirring the first sentiments of independent nationhood. In this context it was possible to discard tradition and generate revolutionary ideas, which Alexander did – motivated by his determination to be an internationally respected star of the theatre. He had had a passionate fascination for Shakespeare since a Scotsman, Robert Robertson (1854–1888), had first introduced him to the sonnets and plays at the age of ten. Young Matthias would look out from the ocean lighthouse in Wynyard, the obscure home of his birth in 1869, wondering how to escape this backward town that had nicknamed him 'mad Fred': 'Oh for a muse of fire, that would ascend the brightest heaven of invention…'

He worked at a tin mine in his home state of Tasmania – three years of clerical work from the age of 16 – until his savings took him to the cosmopolitan shores of Melbourne, where, within a few short months, he began his career as an actor. He was a dynamo and started his own theatre group, held down various jobs, studied the viola and performed. He was beginning to be in demand – and then the gasping breath was brought to his attention. Soon after, he was also getting hoarse.

Despite all this promise and ambition, was Alexander's blossoming career about to be snipped short by an intractable problem of voice loss? This story is told by Alexander in 'Evolution of a Technique', a chapter in his best book, *The Use of the Self.* Starting at this crisis point in his life, he writes:

'The climax came when I was offered a particularly attractive and important engagement [and] I was frankly afraid to accept it.'

He acted on a doctor's advice in the hope that his career could be saved:

'After a few days I felt assured that the doctor's promise would be fulfilled, for I found that by using my voice as little as possible I gradually lost my hoarseness. When the night of the recital came, I was quite free from hoarseness, but before I was halfway through my programme, my voice was in the most distressing condition again, and by the end of the evening the hoarseness was so acute that I could hardly speak.'

A flash of genius

Now came the insight that would eventually elevate Alexander to take his place amongst the profound thinkers of the 20th century. Yet his insight was so simple it was shocking. Like Newton before him who had asked, 'Why did the apple fall?', Alexander reflected on his dilemma and wondered, 'Why is it that when I rest my voice it improves?'

'Is it not fair [he asked his doctor] to conclude that it was something I was doing that evening in using my voice that was the cause of the trouble?'

But what? The doctor did not know and frankly admitted it. He also agreed with Alexander that it was a reasonable theory, one that Alexander quickly put to test by comparing his coordination during speaking to that during reciting in front of a mirror (see heading 'Discovering "backwards and down"' in Chapter 7):

> 'I was particularly struck by three things that I saw myself doing. I saw that as soon as I started to recite, I tended to pull back the head, depress the larynx and suck in breath through the mouth in such a way as to produce a gasping sound.'

This was an encouraging discovery. If he did this during reciting and could manage to stop it, wouldn't his voice then improve? And then Alexander bumped into the first of a long series of perplexing dilemmas that stretched out this period of investigation for ten years, often involving many hours a day of experimental observation in front of mirrors.

A simple experiment

To understand Alexander's initial difficulty, accept this challenge: attempt to rise up out of a chair without tightening your neck or pulling your head back. You may succeed if you deliberately pull your head forward, but that doesn't count – you still tighten your neck. The key here is not to do something new; it is simply to stop doing what you are doing, which is tightening your neck and pulling your head back a little. Try it and see if you do. If you make this experiment honestly, you will find exactly what Alexander found: it can't be done. Or so it seems. In Alexander's case, no matter what he thought, no matter how hard he tried, he found that he could not stop himself from tightening his neck and pulling his head back. What could be done about that?

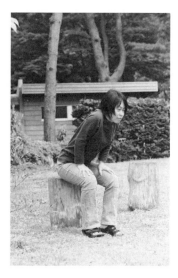

Every time we stand, we almost always tighten
our neck and pull back our head. See if you can
stop doing this. Photo by Akihiro Tada.

In many ways we have all faced this kind of difficulty. We
want to diet, quit drinking or stop eating chocolates, yet,
despite all our good intentions, we, like Alexander, still
keep doing the opposite of what we believe we should be
doing. Alexander was fond of quoting the apostle St Paul's
observation, 'The good thing I want to do I never do; the
evil thing which I do not want – that is what I do' (Romans
7:19). It is a dilemma as old as time itself and heralds the
first inkling of why Alexander's discoveries should continue
to blossom today, over a century after his initial experiments
and more than 50 years since his death.

The methodology

Alexander was a scientist in the 'watch and wonder' class,
an empirical thinker who always insisted that his students

organize their thinking in terms of practice then theory, never theory then practice. It may seem a small point but it lies at the crux of Alexander's approach. He learnt by watching himself, by thinking about what he saw and then finding a reasonable explanation for it.

So he had seen these three tendencies in his mirror. He suspected that these might be a cause of his voice difficulty. Yet now, when he tried to use this information to stop pulling his head back, he couldn't do it. So what could he do now? Instead of being closer to an answer, he was even further from it! What did he do? He just kept watching and wondering. It was what he always did when faced with this first of many problems:

> 'There was nothing for it but to persevere, and I practised patiently month after month, as I had been doing hitherto, with varying experiences of success and failure, but without much enlightenment.'

So, why is it difficult for us to diet, quit drinking or stop eating chocolates? Because that isn't the whole problem; it is only an aspect of it – but it is the aspect we most clearly see. Hidden to our awareness may be deeper causes for our behaviour, causes that are not being addressed in our facile attempts to change. We may overeat because we are lonely, because we find comfort in it; we may smoke because of nerves, or to feel socially at ease; chocolates may rekindle the taste of an earlier, happier time, populated with loving adults who have long since passed from our lives.

A widening search

Alexander's case was no different. He saw that associated with his head and neck being pulled back, his whole body was collapsing down, his shoulders were narrowing and, not only that, all the gestures, expressions and actions associated with his performance were intertwined with the simple action of pulling his head back and down:

> 'Observation in the mirror shewed [sic] me that when I was standing to recite I was using these other parts [arms, legs, gestures] in certain wrong ways which synchronised with my wrong way of using my head and neck, larynx, vocal and breathing organs, and which involved a condition of undue tension throughout my organism.'

This was hopeful. He saw that he had been trying to change just a tiny aspect of what was actually a holistically coordinated action of all his body parts. Of course there was no hope of stopping his head from pulling back when it was actually the movement of shortening his torso that helped to pull it down. He had to change his head and change his torso at the same time, but how should he move his torso? And what's more, how should he move his arms and his legs and how was he going to reduce all the general tension he felt?!

Considering this, it becomes clear why Alexander spent so many years trying to figure all this out. Even in the simple matter of stopping his head from pulling back, he was in a maze:

> 'For where was I to begin? Was it the sucking in of breath that caused the pulling back of the head and the depressing of the larynx? Or was it the pulling back of the head that caused the depressing of the larynx and the sucking in of breath? Or was it the depressing of the larynx that caused the sucking in of breath and the pulling back of the head?'

It was during this long period that Alexander devised the famous 'Alexander directions' which are analyzed in more depth in Chapters 3 and 7.

A shift in paradigms

Yet there was a more profound movement afoot in Alexander's thinking, a revolutionary view totally at odds with the prevailing scientific and philosophical view of the time. When he had started out, he admits that:

> 'I, in common with most people, conceived of "body" and "mind" as separate parts of the same organism, and consequently believed that human ills, difficulties and shortcomings could be classified as either "mental" or "physical" and dealt with on specifically "mental" or specifically "physical" lines.'

However, what his research was showing him now was that all of these complicated coordinated actions of his head, torso, arms and legs could not be dealt with separately as he had been trying to do. He realized that they all came into play instantly in response to a stimulus to speak. There was no one 'part' of him that needed 'fixing', yet this is how he had been thinking of the problem. No wonder he wasn't getting anywhere.

Actually we all still do think like this. We say things like 'I have a sore back' or 'My neck is stiff,' but this kind of thinking, Alexander realized, is delusional as it does not relate to how things actually function. It would be truer to say 'I am a sore back' for that is the truth of the situation. There is no 'back' that is sore separate from who I am.

Alexander realized that he had been thinking in terms of fixing his vocal apparatus, as though that was somehow separate from the rest of him; that he could somehow change this without changing himself. Of course, when you think about it, that is a ridiculous idea. Whenever does your vocal apparatus stop being you? Alexander didn't have a voice problem; he *was* a voice problem! And this meant that he had to change his total reaction before he did anything else.

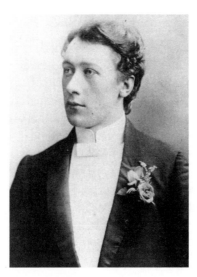

Alexander in 1894. At this time he was already formulating ideas that would prove to be revolutionary for their time.

He christened this 'the critical moment', and henceforth his investigation took on an entirely different flavour. It was a paradigm shift in his thinking, a movement away from the Cartesian universe of neatly separate phenomena, which could be dealt with individually in their turn, to our emerging modern-day view, epitomized by Einstein's Theory of Relativity, that everything, including time and matter itself, are in a constant, shifting relationship; that nothing exists independent of other things; and that a change in one area will cause a change in another. Alexander expresses this idea in his own peculiar, arduous way, when he writes:

> 'It is important to remember that the use of a specific part in any activity is closely associated with the use of other parts of the organism, and that the influence exerted by the various parts one upon the other is

> continuously changing in accordance with the manner
> of use of these parts.'

Shaking one part of a mobile moves every part; none of
it can be considered separate. Modern therapists consider
families the same way. If a child is acting up, they look at
the whole environment of the family for a reason. Is the
child's behaviour a reflection of something else that is going
on? Alexander's conclusion about the body was the same:
you cannot say a problem with, say, a knee is just that; you
must consider the whole context, right up to your head and
neck relationship, to understand your knee problem. But
Alexander was thinking this in the 1890s and at that time
such thoughts were nothing short of revolutionary. He was
way ahead of his time.

Coming to an impasse

By now Alexander had figured out how to coordinate his
body to partially remedy his voice loss. It is worth noting
that, despite his failure to fully implement these discoveries,
he was still achieving some relief from his symptoms. It
was this relief that confirmed he was on the right track –
his experiments were guided by noticing what relieved his
symptoms and what exacerbated them. It was through this
approach of elimination that he slowly came to understand
what he needed to do. This illustrates an important health
principle of the Alexander work: *use affects functioning.*

Alexander had now been experimenting for several years
and, although he was not completely free of hoarseness, his
condition had improved to the point where he was able to
perform confidently again. An ordinary person would no
doubt have stopped at this point and got on with their career.
Not Alexander. He had become intrigued by this whole new
way of thinking:

'I began to see that my findings up till now implied the possibility of the opening up of an entirely new field of inquiry, and I was obsessed with the desire to explore it.'

The problem Alexander was about to confront was his most startling to date. Now that he understood how he must coordinate himself, it was time to put it into practice. He did so, and felt that he was succeeding in doing this, but to his dismay there seemed to be no further improvement in his voice. By his own admission, he'd gotten a little cocky at this stage and had dispensed with his mirrors, thinking that there was nothing more for him to learn. His failure, however, suggested that something was amiss. He tells us:

'This made me suspicious that I was not doing what I thought I was doing, and I decided once more to bring the mirror to my aid… I found that my suspicions were justified. For there I saw that at the critical moment when I tried to combine the prevention of shortening with a positive attempt to maintain a lengthening and speak at the same time, I did not put my head forward and up as I intended, but actually put it back. Here was startling proof that I was doing the opposite of what I believed I was doing and of what I had decided I ought to do.'

This was a big problem. If his feeling told him he was being successful, yet the objective evidence of the mirrors contradicted this, then he was deluding himself. This, as he later discovered during his teaching career, is a universal delusion that we all suffer from.

The universal delusion

This point was brought home to me most clearly by my own teacher, Marjorie Barstow, when she made the simple comment one day: 'You can't reduce tension by making tension.'

When I first heard her say that, I thought, 'Well, that's obvious; there's nothing new in that,' but then I began to observe myself and others and suddenly I realized that making tension is all I ever did in my efforts to reduce it!

Think of yourself: what do you do when your neck feels stiff? Probably, if you're like most people, you pull it down, stretch it, roll it around in a circle or give it a shake – all actions that increase the tension in your neck. How can increasing tension reduce it? How can a stiff neck be made freer by stiffening it further? Does that make sense to you?

Alexander discovered, much to his dismay, that although he *felt* what he was doing was the right thing, it turned out to be the complete opposite. It might feel natural for us to stretch our neck when it's tight, yet, when you stop to think about it, when did that action ever really relieve your tension? Recognizing this delusional aspect of his feelings put Alexander in a real pickle:

> 'This indeed was a blow. If ever anyone was in an impasse, it was I. For here I was, faced with the fact that my feeling, the only guide I had to depend upon for the direction of my use, was untrustworthy.'

Feelings being untrustworthy is not such a strange idea. Neurosis is an example of this same phenomenon that Alexander was encountering in himself. All of us have, at one time or another, come across someone who felt all kinds of things about us, which we knew were simply not true. Intimate relationships form a context where we most often encounter these delusional aspects of feelings.

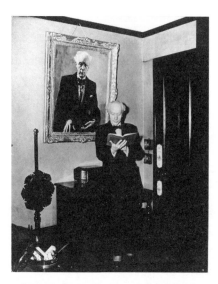

Alexander spent many years watching himself in
the process of reciting to discover how he could
change his coordination and restore his voice.

We describe someone as having 'paranoia' when they falsely
assign negative motives to us. But for the 'paranoid' person,
their feelings are very real. They trust them, act upon them
and, as a result, often cause the very result they most fear. To
be unjustly accused of being angry, for example, can irritate
you to the point of anger!

So what was Alexander to do?

'This led me to a long consideration of the whole
question of the direction of the use of myself. "What is
this direction", I asked myself, "upon which I have been
depending?"'

Direction

Alexander realized that his impulse to move was being driven unconsciously, associated with feelings that had become unreliable. In his mirrors he saw that this impulse occurred almost instantaneously in response to the *idea of reciting*, and the response entailed all the conditions of misuse that he had so meticulously catalogued over the last few years. It wasn't that one little bit of it occurred and the rest was fine; everything happened and it all happened in one instant.

So, through this reasoning:

'I concluded that if I were ever to be able to react satisfactorily to the stimulus to use my voice, I must replace my old instinctive (unreasoned) direction of myself by a new conscious (reasoned) direction.'

What Alexander was trying to do here is a bit like the experience of going overseas and suddenly finding that you have to drive on the opposite side of the road. All your instinctive impulses, if you followed them, could get you killed. It is a strange sensation for, in each moment, you cannot let your instinctive feeling take over and direct your actions; you must instead act consciously. So, in the beginning, you go against your 'feelings' because they have, in this new context, become unreliable.

This was one of Alexander's hobby horses all his life. He maintained that because the world was changing more rapidly than it ever had before, it was becoming increasingly necessary for our healthy survival to be able to re-educate our feelings. You cannot assume that a set of responses developed early in your life can continue to act as a reliable guide for your actions later in life. Most of modern psychology is constructed around this simple premise.

In this regard, Alexander anticipated the explosion in the Western world of the practice of psychoanalysis, psychotherapy and all the other mind-feeling therapies that populate the modern scene. This idea of Alexander's also has its parallels with the psychological concept of transference – where we falsely impute our perceptions towards another based on past experiences. But Alexander was wrestling these concepts while Freud was still writing his 1895 watershed *Project for a Scientific Psychology*. In Sydney, Australia, where Alexander now lived, there was nothing to take refuge in but his own empirical practice:

> 'I set out to put this idea into practice, but I was at once brought up short by a series of startling and unexpected experiences.'

What happened?

He still continued with his old habitual response, despite his now more 'conscious' effort to change. Haven't we all had this experience? How many New Year's resolutions have you been able to keep? Sure, for a few weeks, even for a month or so, we can consciously guide ourselves in our new behaviour: giving up those sweets; arriving on time for appointments; quitting cigarettes; but then some crisis happens and before we know it we are back to our old ways. We keep slipping uncontrollably between the new and the old. This was Alexander's experience too:

> 'In actual practice I found that there was no clear dividing line between my unreasoned and my reasoned direction of myself, and that I was quite unable to prevent the two from overlapping.'

What Alexander did next was quite unexpected: he gave up. He decided he just wouldn't try to do the new thing; he would let it go, separate himself completely from his 'end' and instead devote his attention to the 'means'. This was the birth of another guiding principle of Alexander's discoveries: the concept of 'endgaining'.

Endgaining

We all 'endgain' at one time or another. 'Endgaining' is when we let the idea of what we want so dominate our mind that we fail to pay attention to the means necessary to gain it. A classic example of endgaining is rushing to get somewhere. In our rush we often cause accidents which delay our departure.

For example, I may be trying to finish the dishes quickly before my favourite TV show starts, but because I worry so much, half-watching the television in the other room, I fail to notice a glass on the table and knock it over. Now it's going to take me even longer. Had I paid full attention to what I was doing – which is, after all, the only real means to accomplishing my goal of finishing the dishes in time – I would not have knocked the glass over and could have finished earlier.

Endgaining is a way of life for some people, but it comes at a terrible cost. Heart attacks, anxiety attacks, injuries and general stress all result from this kind of living. In sports, endgaining can mean death. If a racing driver loses his attention for even a second, it can be fatal.

Being obsessed with winning is OK, provided it doesn't impair our attentiveness on the field. Greedy ambition, however, can distort our view – by letting the obsession overtake our mind and thus losing concentration on the task at hand. *We have to let go of the idea of winning in order to win.* In this case, 'letting go of winning' could mean giving up the anxiety of losing. After all, you wouldn't be anxious about losing if winning didn't mean a lot to you, would you? But if you take that anxiety on to the field of play, it can be potentially lethal to your chances of winning.

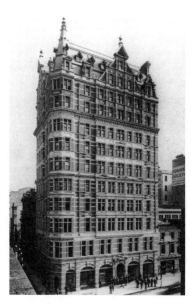

It was in this building in Melbourne that Alexander began
to discover 'endgaining': when our attention is only on
the result, we are unable to see *how* we do something.

This is the devious mechanism of 'endgaining' as Alexander
conceived it. He had to give up the idea of getting what he
wanted, because it was getting in the way of him getting
what he wanted. The further we progress into Alexander's
story, the trickier the concepts start to be, for now he was
exploring the very nature of the mind, and not only of mind
but the important, inter-dependent relationship that mind
has with feelings. He comments:

> 'For I saw that an immediate response was the result of
> a decision on my part to do something at once, to go
> directly for a certain end, and by acting quickly on this
> decision I did not give myself the opportunity to project
> as many times as was necessary the new directions which

I had reasoned out were the best means whereby I could attain this end.'

This new insight into his behaviour was extraordinary. Alexander was telling himself, in effect, that the only way he could gain what he wanted was to stop wanting it!

When I first came into contact with the 12 steps of the Alcoholics Anonymous programme, I was initially taken by the similarity of their first step and Alexander's approach. Both advocate that the way to change is to give up the desperate effort of trying to be in control of your end. You give up, for example, the idea that you have the power to control your alcoholic consumption. The alcoholic might think to himself, 'I can stop drinking whenever I want to – I just choose not to,' but the first step in AA says, 'We admitted that we were powerless over alcohol and that our lives had become unmanageable.'

Accepting ourselves

It always struck me as odd that the first step of a programme whose explicit aim is to guide you into sobriety by giving up alcohol asks you to admit, as its first step, that you have no power over alcohol! What lies under this step, and Alexander's own realization at this stage of his investigation, is self-acceptance.

If the motivation to change is driven by an aversion to what I do, then to change I always need the energy of this aversion: a paradox that cannot be resolved by greater effort, for the greater the effort, the greater the aversion must become. Alexander remarked about this strange phenomenon of human behaviour:

'Trying is only emphasizing the thing we already know.'

He realized that:

> '…it would be necessary for me to make the experience of receiving the stimulus to speak and of refusing to do anything immediately in response.'

The key phrase here is 'to make the experience'. This means breaking your mind's link between the person you want to be and the person you are. Why should this be so important?

As they discovered in the 12-step programme, the problem centres around self-acceptance. If you are constantly trying to be that which you are not, you don't experience yourself as you are. In the AA programme it is necessary to admit, 'I am an alcoholic.' In Alexander's programme it is necessary to give up wanting your end and say, 'This is how I am.' Alexander said:

> 'People that haven't any fish to fry, they see it all right.'

Thinking in activity

But if you give up gaining your end, what do you do instead? What was Alexander going to do if he wasn't going to speak? Just stand there and do nothing? That's right. That's exactly what he did. He writes that he spent 'long periods together, for successive days and weeks and sometimes even months'.

He was doing nothing else but standing in front of his mirrors and giving himself the directions to change his coordination. Imagine what this meant: hours of silent observation of himself, months of quietly standing and bringing into play the directions of his use. The inspiration for the 'Primary holding pattern' process described in Chapter 6 comes from this practice of Alexander's. It is not unlike the practice of some forms of meditation.

Professor John Dewey, Alexander's good friend and long-time pupil, described this process as 'thinking in activity' and Alexander claims that:

> '...anyone who carries it out faithfully while trying to gain an end will find that he is acquiring a new experience in what he calls "thinking".'

This is the point when words become entirely inadequate in describing Alexander's voyage of discovery, for he fundamentally discovered a way of imparting a new experience and it can no more be described than a kiss can be posted.

Thinking in activity is a process of projecting a number of different directions together in their sequence. In Alexander jargon, it's called 'giving your directions'. What are these directions that must be given? This is the essence of an Alexander lesson: a teacher is trained to impart the experience of these different directions through the use of his or her hands. Each direction is designed to guide your nervous system back towards an integrated and efficient pattern of coordination. These directions are the result of Alexander's extended period of research into his, and by implication, all human coordination. All this is explained in greater length in Chapters 3 and 7.

The critical moment

Eventually, the time had to come when Alexander sought to apply his new 'thinking in activity' process in speaking. Now he was to meet the last and mightiest obstacle yet in his decade-long odyssey:

> 'The time came when I believed that I had practised the "means whereby" enough, and I started to employ them

for the purpose of speaking, but to my dismay I found that I failed far more often than I succeeded.'

What was wrong? Alexander had no idea. He writes:

'The fact remained that I failed more often than not, and nothing was more certain than that I must go back and reconsider my premises.'

He carefully reasoned out again that the directions he was giving himself were the right ones. He had no doubt of that. So, given that that wasn't the problem, he investigated other possibilities – even questioning whether this was a case of his own unique inadequacies.

His attention centred again on the critical moment. Having become familiar with the experience of thinking in activity, he felt that he was continuing with this throughout the activity, yet it wasn't working. He writes:

'I came to the conclusion that it was necessary for me to seek some concrete proof whether, at the critical moment when I attempted to gain my end and speak, I was really continuing to project the directions in their proper sequence for the employment of the new and more satisfactory use, as I thought I was, or whether I was reverting to the instinctive misdirection of my old habitual use which had been associated with all my throat trouble.'

Guess what he found? He wasn't doing it. But why?

This was the tough question and Alexander's answer to it was inspired. By careful experimentation, it dawned on him that parallel with the process of 'giving' his directions was another process of 'feeling' his directions, and it was this secondary process that was disrupting his attempt to coordinate himself differently to speak.

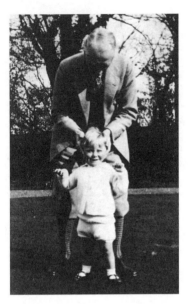

Even children can develop the kind of misuse that
had almost crippled Alexander's acting career.

My teacher Marjorie Barstow used to say, 'You think,
you move and then you feel', but what Alexander now
discovered was that he had it all around the wrong way.
He was thinking, then feeling and then moving. But what
were his feelings looking for? They were looking for the
experience that felt right and natural, and it suddenly hit
Alexander that the experience he actually wanted would feel
totally wrong. How could it be otherwise?

As he often pointed out to others, you can't change and
stay the same while you do it, but that was exactly what he
was trying to do. Alexander argued to himself that if the way
he coordinated himself habitually was what felt normal to
him, then didn't it follow that any new way would not feel
normal, even feel completely wrong? Of course it would, he
realized. Yet here he was, giving unfamiliar directions while

seeking out an accompanying feeling to do them that felt familiar:

> 'I now had to face the fact that in all my attempts during these past months I had been trying to employ a new use of myself which was bound to feel wrong, at the same time trusting to my feeling of what was right to tell me whether I was employing it or not.'

Small wonder that this attempt had proved futile! In AA they call it 'Letting go and letting God'. Alexander was never a religious man – in fact, he once ruffled a few Christian feathers with his opinion that Jesus had great teachings but was poor on technique – but Alexander's discovery of how to make a real change is profound.

The nature of change

To truly make a change, we enter into a new world where all that was familiar is gone. And we can't hold on to the past while we are living out the future. Alexander discovered that 'holding on' to what felt familiar left him unable to experience the unfamiliar.

If he did let go and follow his new directions, it felt odd. Alexander lessons feel odd. A pupil of mine once joked that after his Alexander lessons it took him 30 minutes to remember his name. I know what he means – Alexander lessons have the capacity to reach deep into the terrain of your 'self', clearing away a lot of obstructions in your psychological landscape. It is possible to experience a you that is tucked away and hidden, a you different from the person you imagine yourself to be and closer to the person you are. In that sense, Alexander lessons can be profound and quite scary.

Survivors of abuse have told many stories of reawakening to terrors of the past as the protective layers of tension dissolved away through their Alexander lessons. As Alice Miller once expressed it:

> The truth about our childhood is stored up in our body, and although we can repress it, we can never alter it. Our intellect can be deceived, our feelings manipulated, our perceptions confused, and our body tricked by medication. But someday the body will present its bill, for it is as incorruptible as a child who, still whole in spirit, will accept no compromises or excuses, and it will not stop tormenting us until we stop evading the truth.

Conclusion

Not all Alexander lessons are this profound; much of that depends on the skill and nature of your teacher, which I have discussed in Chapter 4. In Alexander's case, all he sought was to fix his voice and get back to the stage. However, he didn't get back, for his new discovery turned out to be the final piece that completed the puzzle.

Alexander now had a plan. And a plan that worked. A good teacher can quickly familiarize you with this plan. It involves making a choice. Alexander tells us that he would make a decision to speak, then give himself the experience of refusing to speak. At that critical moment he would again give his directions and consider his options. Maybe he would speak. Maybe he would lift an arm. Maybe he would do nothing, other than continuing with the process of giving himself directions. He writes:

> 'After I had worked on this plan for a considerable time, I became free from my tendency to revert to my wrong habitual use in reciting, and the marked effect of this upon my functioning convinced me that I was at last on the right track, for once free of this tendency, I also

become free from the throat and nasal difficulties with which I had been beset from birth.'

And others could see that, somehow, there had been a remarkable change in Alexander, and soon people were asking him, 'How did you do it? Can you teach me?' While in New Zealand, on one of the last of his serious acting tours (he did appear at the Old Vic in London as Shylock in *The Merchant of Venice*), a group of his pupils wrote and begged that he continue his teaching instead of resuming his acting career. Upon his return to Australia, he considered their request seriously.

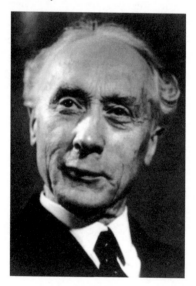

Not only did Alexander restore his own voice but he created a new one; a voice that now, more than 50 years after his death in 1955, continues to be heard further and farther afield.

The fateful moment came one summer's day in 1903. Alexander hopped on a tram in Melbourne whereupon he accidentally met his bookie who offered him odds of

150:1 on a race to be run later that day. Forever a risk-taker, Alexander laid on a bet of five pounds – a small fortune in those days – and won.

The wild isolation of Australia had thrown up this remarkable man, but in 1903 London was at the centre of the world and Alexander knew it. He took his money and sailed off, arriving on the shores of England in 1904. He never returned. The boy from Wynyard certainly achieved his fame, but not as the actor he had longed to be. Instead, he far surpassed even his own dreams by creating a system that today is employed by almost every major performing arts institution in the Western world. There's hardly an actor alive today who hasn't heard of him. Not only did Alexander restore his own voice but he created a new one; a voice that now, more than half a century after his death in 1955, continues to be heard further and farther afield.

3

Physiology of Movement

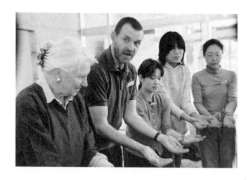

'They may teach you anatomy and physiology till they are black in the face – you will still have this to face, sticking to a decision against the habit of life.'

F. M. Alexander

I work a lot with actors, and during my first lesson with them I demonstrate how powerfully they are 'characterized' by their patterns of coordination. We all carry or 'hold' ourselves together in a particular way, and our bigger movements are then influenced by this underlying 'carrying' action as shown with the characters in Figure 3.1. Alexander said:

'Talk about a man's individuality and character: it's the way he uses himself.'

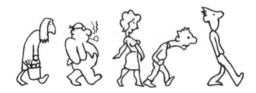

Figure 3.1 Alexander: 'Talk about a man's individuality
and character: it's the way he uses himself.'

This 'self' we love to talk about is, in physiological terms,
a hypothetical entity. While supposedly driving our actions,
a 'self' cannot be found in our bodily systems in the same
way that our heart, liver or brain can be found. Our 'self'
arises out of a vastly complicated set of responses which
themselves are caused by a variety of causes and conditions
in our environment; put them all together and a 'self'
is implied, but it exists as a collection of learnt responses
to certain conditions, conditions which themselves are
changing on a moment-to-moment basis. This is lucky for
us because it implies that we can change previously learnt
responses to certain conditions and in that way change our
'self'. Alexander's third book was called *The Use of the Self.*

This chapter is an exploration of that 'self' as it arises
in our movement physiology – which is the study of the
processes of our body and mind. This is a vast subject, a
little like trying to analyze matter. You can go as far as atoms
and it all seems quite neat and logical. Go any further into a
subatomic realm and you meet quantum theory and quarks,
and all logic quickly falls apart.

Studying the physiology of movement is a little like that.
There's a level where it makes sense, yet there's a deeper
level where everything seems to be affecting everything else
and every statement about how something works has to be
qualified by 20 others, because a hundred different things

could change it. I am not going introduce you to all those 'qualifications' because I don't understand it myself.

The title of this chapter is deceptive for I do not offer a total picture of our movement physiology. To do so would easily fill a whole book. I am going leave out a lot of information and still be simplistic about what I do include, maybe a little too much so, but my aim is not to help you pass an exam – go to university for that – but to offer some ideas that are useful *practically* when setting about making changes to your movement patterns.

Motor hold and motor move

The most intriguing idea in movement physiology, from our point of view, is the organization of both muscles and neural networks (the wiring) into what physiologists call the 'motor hold' and 'motor move' systems.

When you stand up straight, why is it that you don't collapse in a heap on the floor? Because certain muscles, called the intrinsic muscles, 'hold' you together. These muscles are short, taut and busy nearly all the time. They lie at the deepest level, close to the bone itself, and are involved in whatever we are doing – that is why their technical name is the 'intrinsic' muscles. I call them 'the being muscles' because they help you to 'be' standing. The collective name for all these muscles and the neural networks responsible for their organization and function is the 'motor hold' system.

When you decide to move, another whole set of muscles is brought into play. These muscles, called the extrinsic muscles, are longer, stronger and lie more superficially – closer to the skin than the skeleton. The aesthetic curves of the human body are formed by these large, powerful muscles and they are chiefly involved in making the larger movements – such as walking, waving, bending. So for these reasons their technical name is the 'extrinsic' muscles, but I will call them the 'doing' muscles because they 'do' all the big movements. The collective name for all these muscles and the neural networks responsible for their organization and function is the 'motor move' system.

Being and doing muscles

You couldn't really tell the difference if you looked at these two kinds of muscles under a microscope – although there are some differences which I will get to later – because this classification is more functional than structural – that is, it is how we use them that defines their category. For this reason a muscle can sometimes be classed as both a 'being' and 'doing' muscle because it can perform either role. Sometimes a muscle acts to stabilize a movement, other times to make a movement. What happens if we 'misuse' them, if we make them do the opposite of what they were designed to do?

Take, for example, running. Some people seem to wobble about in a careless fashion, wasting a lot of energy and effort to make movements, such as bobbing their heads up and down and twisting their body from side to side, that contribute nothing to their running – except perhaps to slow it down.

This is an example of 'doing' muscles working unnecessarily. The Olympians, however, run as smooth as the wind itself, focusing every inch of their effort toward that primary goal of speed, eliminating all unnecessary movements. Only those muscles that need to do *do*, while the rest are carefully *being* – that is, creating a stable structure around which the limbs can make their magic.

It is important that the division of labour between these two muscle types is accomplished satisfactorily; otherwise, all sorts of problems start to crop up. One of the worst is collapse: we find we can no longer be comfortable sitting upright. We continuously slump – not only while sitting in a chair, which isn't necessarily a bad thing of itself (after all, cats slump too), but *all the time.*

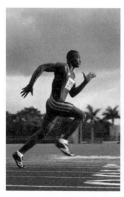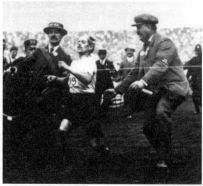

These two photos illustrate dramatically the difference in coordination between two runners. The runner on the left illustrates that the Olympians run as smooth as the wind itself, focusing every inch of their effort toward that primary goal of speed, eliminating all unnecessary movements. The photograph on the right, which shows Dorando completing a marathon race in London in 1908, was published in Alexander's first book, *Man's Supreme Inheritance*, as an example of needless, uncontrolled exertion. Notice how this runner leans backwards, not forward, to complete the race. (See *MSI*, Part 2, Chapter 7.)

We slump while we walk, slump to get in or out of a chair, slump to pick something up. Eventually, we can never get comfortable. We always feel tired and have aches in our body and it becomes a great weight, a burden to live in. We know that continuous slumping is unhealthy for us, but sitting up seems like a great effort too and, in many ways, seems even more of a strain than slumping. Either way, we always feel sore and tired. Why?

Part of the answer lies in the way muscles consume energy. And that is a result of the job they have to do. The being muscles of the motor hold system work very hard – they almost never stop – whereas the doing muscles of the motor move system are only called upon to contract from time to time; they momentarily rest between the execution of one movement and the next.

The poor old being muscles, however, have a really hard time of it; even lying flat on your back asleep requires muscular activity. Without it, other systems such as breathing, digestion and circulation could be adversely affected. However, during sleep few of the larger doing muscle movements need to occur – maybe to roll over now and again but not that much more. So while the doing muscles always have time to rest, the being muscles have almost none. To accommodate these two kinds of demands, there are two kinds of muscle fibre: red muscle fibre and white muscle fibre.

Fatigable and non-fatigable muscle fibres

A muscle fibre is a muscle cell and they come in two varieties: red and white. White muscle fibres are also called fatigable muscle fibres. If you use a white muscle fibre for a long time, it will fatigue – there will be a build-up of chemicals that eventually cause so much pain that you aren't willing to sustain the contraction. Red muscle fibres, however, because of the special way they burn energy, can be contracted your entire life without any such pain; hence they are also known as non-fatigable muscle fibres. While every muscle contains both kinds of fibre, one structural factor that does distinguish between a doing and a being muscle is how much of each kind of fibre is within a given muscle (see Figure 3.2).

A muscle is a collection of millions of these muscle fibres and every muscle contains a higher proportion of one kind of fibre, depending upon the kind of work it is called to do. Can you guess which kind of fibre is more prominent in a being muscle? These intrinsic (motor hold) being muscles obviously contain a high percentage of the red non-fatigable muscle fibres, whereas the extrinsic (motor move) doing muscles contain a larger proportion of the white fatigable muscle fibres.

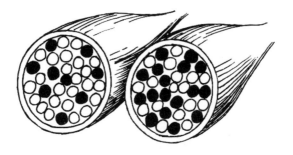

Figure 3.2 This cross-section of both an extrinsic (left) and intrinsic (right) muscle shows the difference in composition of red muscle fibres (dark spots) and white muscle fibres (white spots).

This physiology lays the basis for athletic performance: the great sprinters will have a much higher percentage of the white fatigable muscle fibres to call upon, whereas the great long-distance runners have a much higher percentage of the red non-fatigable fibres. To a certain extent, their athletic fate was genetically predetermined. You rarely, if ever, find athletes who excel at both.

So, returning to the question posed earlier, why do we get sore and tired and want to slump all the time? In our daily life we can come to use the fatigable fibres to do the work that the non-fatigable fibres are better suited to. When that happens, suddenly the white fatigable fibres are being asked to do work normally handled by the red non-fatigable fibres. Trying to 'sit up' by pulling in your lower back and forcefully lifting your chest is an example of this. Obviously, these fatigable fibres don't perform this kind of task well, so we tire easily, get sore muscles and find ourselves slumping almost continuously. Over our life this unabated shortening of our torso progressively affects our whole bodily structure and movement capability, as shown in Figure 3.3.

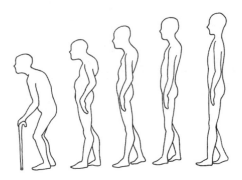

Figure 3.3 The continuous slumping and slouching of our everyday life has a dramatic long-term effect on our structure and movement flexibility.

As well as affecting our movement flexibility, this continuous condition of collapse also places added strain on other systems in the body. For example, a compressed, shortened torso will result in shorter, shallower breathing. Instead of quiet, deep, long breaths, our breathing cycle accelerates towards panting – to get the same amount of air we now have to work harder at it. This effect is mirrored in other systems: blood pressure may increase, our heart rate can rise, even digestion becomes more problematic.

This is information that has yet to be proved conclusively, but my experience as an Alexander teacher tells me that this is true. As a person restores the right balance between the two systems of motor hold and motor move, there are immediate, observable differences – for example, in the nature of breathing.

If you take lessons, you will be able to make proof of this for yourself. There is also an enormous body of anecdotal evidence from the many hundreds of thousands of people who have experienced such benefits during the century that Alexander's discoveries have been spreading.

A healthy condition within our movement system is a prerequisite for optimal functioning of the other bodily systems. While all of them can and do work under any conditions, they will function more efficiently when our movement system is performing well.

Recruitment

From the foregoing you can see that it becomes very important to recruit the right fibre for the right job. Here we meet another concept in the physiology of movement: 'recruitment'. This describes the processes that the nervous system utilizes to appropriately – or inappropriately – 'recruit' the right kind of fibres for the given job.

How well does your nervous system 'recruit' at the moment? Try this little experiment to test the acuity of your own 'recruitment'. Hold your arm out to the side so that your hand is level with your shoulder. Leave it there as you read on. Normally, this activity is accomplished by the larger, doing muscles which are predominantly comprised of the powerful but more easily fatigable white fibres. 'Fatigable' means that your arm is probably starting to feel a little sore. Leave it there longer if it isn't – it will eventually! The thing is, holding your arm out like that is a bit abnormal but it can happen in life – painting a roof, for instance. It's a perfect example of why, tucked in there amongst all those fatigable fibres, are a few non-fatigable ones, which must now be 'recruited' if you will ever be able to continue keeping your arm up. Not many readers will still be holding up their arm without pain, but if you are, congratulations. Your recruitment is excellent. You can put it down now.

Alexander lessons improve recruitment. Any activity that has you focus attention on your movements and encourages delicacy, lightless and ease will facilitate better recruitment. Maladjusted coordination could be defined by saying that there is poor recruitment: white fatigable muscle fibres are trying to do the work of the red non-fatigable muscle fibres which in turn are doing very little – even though they are capable of doing a lot. The coordinated response of our body is no longer harmonious. It's as though every musician in the symphony suddenly decided to play their own tune, creating a cacophony of noise that is totally lacking in harmony. Watch people walking down the street for an hour – their limbs, hips and heads bobbing about every which way or held in an unnecessarily tight fashion – and you'll quickly understand that this description is not as far-fetched as it seems.

But now comes the big question: how can Alexander work improve 'recruitment'?

Inhibition as freedom

To answer this question we need to understand 'inhibition'. As a term used by physiologists, it has nothing to do with the meaning ascribed to it by Freud – far from being about repression, our idea of inhibition concerns freedom. Although it was Sherrington who made the important discovery of inhibitory neurons in the nervous system, it could be argued that the discovery of the *principle* of inhibition in controlling everyday movement was equally Alexander's – it is the essence of the Alexander approach.

Alexander was one of the world's great physiologists. He may not have known all the long Latin names or have been able to describe microscopic activity in the neuromuscular system, but he knew more about the practical matter of movement control in a holistic sense than any of his contemporaries. The common view that is held – the view that physiologists once held – is that excitation is the only means of controlling movement. We want to do something; we contract our muscles and do it, end of story. But it isn't quite like that and this was the first fundamental discovery Alexander made in the realm of human behaviour: that 'inhibition', as well as 'excitation', is an essential ingredient in the control of movement, as shown in Figure 3.4.

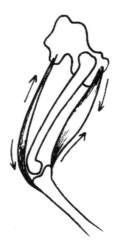

Figure 3.4 When we bend our leg, we obviously excite muscles to contract (shown by the arrows pointing towards each other) but we must also inhibit the activity of an opposing set of muscles (shown by the arrows pointing away from each other) for the leg to be able to bend.

This is the first and primary point to understand about Alexander 'directions', which will be discussed at length in Chapter 7. They are not designed to excite muscles to achieve a specific result – as happens when we make movements normally; instead, they are designed to inhibit or prevent the continuation of a result that is already underway!

Read that sentence again – it is critical to understanding everything that follows. It is the 'inhibition' of inappropriate activity that is the order of the day, not the excitation of new activity. In Alexander jargon, this concept goes under the name of 'non-doing', which can be roughly equated with 'inhibition'.

Inhibition exists at a cellular level and then at ascending levels of organization in the nervous system right up to, and including, full cortical or voluntary control. Let's start at a cellular level and follow the action upwards, remembering that we are working towards an understanding of how 'inhibition' will improve the 'recruitment' of our red and white muscle fibres within both our intrinsic and extrinsic musculature in order to improve the functioning of all our bodily systems.

Motor neurons: inhibition and excitation

A motor neuron is a little device – a biological cell, in fact – that shoots out a charge that will either contract a muscle or inhibit that contraction. Neurons that excite are called, not surprisingly, 'excitory' motor neurons, and the other kind are 'inhibitory' motor neurons.

You realize why you need these 'inhibitory' neurons when you consider that at a primitive level our brain is always trying to make every movement it can. Our muscular system is being bombarded with an awesome outpouring of neuro-electric impulses which could, if it weren't for higher brain centres 'inhibiting' some of these messages, throw our body into a crisis of spasm, utterly immobilizing our movement. You have seen people suffer from this lack of inhibition, their arms and legs contracting in ways beyond their control because of damage sustained by their nervous system.

While we all have these impulses flooding down through our spinal cord every second, luckily most of us also have many inhibitory impulses that can counteract this massive excitation – that is the way we organize a coordinated concert of activity. But it seems a little odd, doesn't it, to have all this excitation and then to have to inhibit half of it?

The consequences of this are best summarized by Alexander's observation that the right thing does itself, that 'To know when we are wrong is all that we shall ever know in this world.'

The right thing does itself

It isn't necessary to know how to walk; it is only necessary to know how not to. Control is in process, not superimposed – we are merely directing the force; we are not originating it. You are turning the steering wheel, not pushing the car.

To borrow from a popular sci-fi movie, 'The force is with you'. It never left. It was always there and will always be there. Our problem is that we have 'smothered' it with complex sets of 'pseudo-movements' which forcefully suppress the natural order which is struggling for supremacy – it is this natural order that 'does itself' if we learn to 'inhibit' the wrong thing.

Another useful analogy to understand this key point is to imagine a mirror covered by mud. The mirror still retains the ability to reflect but, outwardly, it appears to be lost. Clear away the mud and the reflection seems to 'reappear'. Actually, it was never not there in the first place. That's how it is with graceful, easy coordination. It seems to be lost and in its place we have stiff necks, tense heavy bodies and many disorders within other systems of our organism. But all that is just mud on the mirror. As Alexander once advised a pupil:

'Like a good fellow, stop the things that are wrong first.'

Yet so much advice to 'improve posture' that is given out today by practitioners of all kinds goes against this basic fact of our physiology. We are told that we have to try to 'correct' our coordination, to 'put' ourselves right by harmful activities such as pulling our shoulders back, tucking in our tails or holding up our chests. This kind of approach is barbaric. All we are doing, by increasing the tension in our bodies, is spreading more mud on the mirror! If we can just stop all the unnecessary and harmful contractions, the underlying pattern is able to re-emerge. Our nervous system doesn't have to learn how to coordinate us well – it already knows it. We just get in its way.

One of the things our nervous system 'knows' is how to bring about appropriate recruitment of fatigable and non-fatigable muscles fibres – again, this is wired in, is already there, is able to reassert itself if we would just let it. So correct recruitment will naturally result if we are able to identify and inhibit those patterns of coordination that we have developed that are both inappropriate and downright harmful. But aren't you wondering, why did we go wrong in the first place? If our movement system is so 'already knowing', why does it continue to guide us incorrectly? Why is it being 'smothered'?

We smother it with our 'self'.

The hypothetical 'self'

The thing that most interferes with our movement development is this hypothetical entity (from a physiologist's point of view) of a 'self'. The exact location of this 'self' has yet to be defined – it may be more the province of religion than physiology – but, in our physiology, it nevertheless has a profound impact on how we develop movement patterns. It is this 'self' that causes most of the problems.

As a toddler, because we are not yet strongly identified with a 'self', there is less chance of interfering with our movement mechanisms. Without the clear sense of identity that we have as adults, let alone opinions, beliefs and the like, a child's cortical or higher brain centres won't interfere with the development of their coordination. At this time the only thing that can harmfully influence their movement development is the model they use to learn from.

We learn to walk because we see our parents doing it. There was a case of a child raised exclusively by wolves who, instead of walking, got around on his hands and feet just like his 'wolf' parents. The models placed before a toddler will profoundly influence their walk. That children move like their parents is not so much genetic as it is an acquired behaviour, as illustrated in Figure 3.5. The toddler's unique pattern of movement is still assembled from components put together at a primitive level in their nervous system.

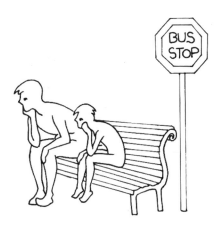

Figure 3.5 As children we unconsciously mimic our parents.

Reflexes and programmes of coordination

Some of our movement patterns are so primitive that we could yank our brain out and they would still work – for a while at least. Walking is not a primitive 'reflex' activity that 'does itself' without the effort of learning. Walking is a complicated movement consisting of many levels of coordinated activity. It does, however, involve the use of primitive reflexes. In physiology, 'reflex' has a definite meaning, subtly different from its everyday usage which I won't explain here – it is too complex for our needs.

Instead, let me make an analogy with something more familiar to you – a classical concerto. In this example, the 'concerto' is a metaphor for our 'walk'. Like walking, it is an immensely complicated thing but, if analyzed, it can be broken down into movements, each movement comprising different sections, and the sections comprising themes which are combinations of melodies and chords. Melodies consist of series of notes in a particular order, and chords are notes played in specific combinations, and, usually, melodies and chords are played together. Every single part of the concerto consists of notes. Nearly everything has chords and melodies. Themes reoccur in different movements, and movements will also, as a whole, have different speeds: 'allegro' or 'adagio'. Complicated, isn't it?

Walking is organized a little like that – involving primitive, automatic reflexes, analogous to the 'notes' of a concerto, right up to the different speeds of a movement, such as skipping, hopping, running. All of these are variations on the theme of walking. Within these movements will be sections – the lifting of one leg followed by the lifting of another combined with the maintenance of an upright stance. Then any one of these actions will have within it different 'melodies' and 'chords'; for example, one person will turn out their foot further on one side. Another person will twist more to the left. These differences are themes that repeat themselves in other movements.

A theme might, for instance, have all the information of how to move my hand to my hair so that everyone who watches it thinks I look very fussy. Another theme may be moving my hand to my hair so that everyone thinks I'm a real slob. However, both movements consist of very similar 'notes' and 'chords' – that is, there are smaller sections that can be assembled to create original, complex movements, and that is where the higher centres of the nervous system come into their own.

We don't control the minutiae of these sections consciously; we just organize them in our own fashion, adding our person. We are born able to execute all the chords and notes that these activities are constructed from; our job is to learn to put them together in the right combinations.

For example, placing the full weight of our body on our foot will mechanically cause a stretch along the fibres of some muscles in our foot. This in turn sets off a reaction called a 'stretch reflex'. It's like turning on a charge: the weight of the foot sets off the 'charge', and the 'charge' becomes the meat that feeds further reactions, rippling right up the body to our head and neck. The end result will be that our extensors maintain our upright stance. But that is a really simple thing compared to what must happen for us to be able to walk.

To walk invokes a whole system of trial and error which is run at a higher level of organization in our nervous system. But the higher the level at which we are constructing, the more opportunity we have to influence how these combinations are put together. A primary source of our potential to 'misuse' is that the models we are mimicking are themselves inefficient.

Mimicking parents is a deliberate action on the part of a child. Walking does not require a twist to the right, but if a child sees this in his mother, he will add such a twist. These coordination patterns sit at the heart of who we think we are and are the most difficult to change. The primary holding pattern of our being muscles can be set with a permanent twist during this time which then forms the basis of everything that follows.

Emotional patterns of coordination

Modern psychotherapeutic theory suggests that our muscles store emotion, and on the basis of that premise many body-workers seek to liberate this stored emotion, releasing thoughts and feelings long held in the muscles of the body. The aspect of our body that is holding this emotion can be equated to the being muscles, and the character themes that emerge (see Figure 3.1) create our personality.

Also, if our models are poor, we get a lousy start and it doesn't stop as a toddler. As we get older and start developing a stronger identity, erroneous ideas begin forming which in turn direct our bodily movements. A woman I worked with had large breasts and a constant, searing pain in her back from trying to push her breasts down and hide their size. Until she was able to hold the thought of accepting her large breasts and not hiding them – which initially produced intense emotional discomfort for her – the pain persisted. As soon as she accepted them, the pain vanished and a blushing new feeling arose.

Another example: we might think we are too tall so we try to make our body shorter. This action, arising out of a desired but delusional self-image, gives rise to a whole range of harmful movement programmes that both interfere with, and end up dominating our underlying balance. Suddenly, our musculature is being asked to conform to a hypothetical body that our 'self' has manufactured. I believe that this is a uniquely human phenomenon – I don't imagine there are too many 'I'm-too-tall' cats wandering about the city.

In this way, we continue adding, twisting, contorting, lifting and generally trying to reshape and protect ourselves – particularly if we are living in an emotionally unsupportive or abusive environment. Some people have a permanent pattern of coordination to 'cower'. You also often see dogs with this kind of look. It was once an appropriate response in violent circumstances but now, long after that emotional environment has altered, it is being perpetuated by becoming its own cause through projecting its expectations on to others. We get trapped by this habituated 'cowering' response until, after many years, this unnecessary pseudo-reaction starts causing physical (and mental) problems we can no longer ignore.

Alexander lessons seek to bring to you a conscious awareness of these pseudo-reactions as they manifest as movements so that you can release them. To try to do even more – by making efforts, for example, to stand tall – is never the way to remedy such a problem. A person needs to give up the habit of cowering, not develop yet another habit of trying not to cower!

Alexander said:

> '…instead of making the decision not to do it, you try to prevent yourself from doing it. But this only means that you decide to do it, and then use muscle tension to prevent yourself from doing it.'

Our underlying pattern of coordination is never lost; it has been imposed upon, so much so that the distorting habits block out all the messages that keep seeking a return to balanced coordination. It is by making this decision 'not to do it' that inhibition forms the heart of any attempt to restore ourselves into balance.

Alexander work is an odd mixture of preventing an unnecessary activity while directing yourself towards a restoration. The 'directions' that Alexander devised are simply descriptions of how our body will coordinate itself when left alone to do it – and these will spontaneously arise when our hypothetical 'self' stops interfering! Ironically, this very 'self', while being a primary cause of our difficulties, also becomes the key to finding our way out again.

If you had to re-read that last paragraph, perhaps it is time to describe an Alexander lesson. In the next chapter I will give you an overview of how a lesson works: the different methods teachers use; how to go about choosing a teacher; and how to decide what works for you.

4

An Alexander Lesson

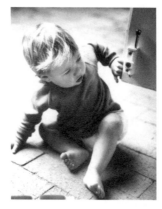

'When an investigation comes to be made it will
be found that every single thing we are doing in
the work is exactly what is being done in Nature
where the conditions are right, the difference
being that we are learning to do it consciously!'

F. M. Alexander

There are three reasons why people take lessons. First, and
by far the most common, is the need to heal: it may be
because of a bad back, a repetitive strain injury or just plain
stress and tension. Second, it may be for professional reasons:
musicians, actors, singers, athletes and others pursuing
excellence have found Alexander lessons an invaluable aid
to their craft. Third, people come for self-improvement: they
are aware that they lack poise, they feel clumsy and awkward

with their bodies and want to improve their carriage and sense of confidence.

Your clarity of purpose and strength of motivation are key factors that determine the success of your lessons. That, and the teacher you choose to go to. Whatever reasons you have for taking lessons, it is extremely important that you find the right teacher. Not every teacher suits every person because we are all different – can everyone be your friend?

In Chapter 5 I have outlined some of the different teaching lineages that have descended from Alexander. This will help a little in making your decision, but, in the end, what really matters is the person, not the teaching style.

A second point to consider is that many Alexander teachers trained later in life so they often have another professional skill. For example, many musicians get into trouble, find Alexander work and end up training as teachers. It could happen to you. If you are a musician, it makes sense to go to a teacher who understands the demands of your craft. I was an actor before I trained, so I specialize in the unique problems actors face in characterization. Other teachers are horse riders, athletes, counsellors and so on, so it's worth enquiring about a teacher's background, especially when faced with a choice.

Alexander teachers will give you a first lesson with no further commitment – if they don't, I wouldn't go to them. During that first lesson you will have an opportunity to discuss your situation, determine costs, frequency and overall number of lessons as well as any anticipated results. You also have a chance to assess whether you feel comfortable with the teacher and their work. Let's look in more detail at each of these points.

Choosing a teacher

Alexander work is very personal, even intimate.

The teacher will learn a great deal about you while you won't learn much about them. Not that you are going to be asked to talk about personal things – Alexander teachers aren't counsellors; they're educators – but the nature of a lesson goes to the essence of your outlook and approach to life. You're there to change the habits of a lifetime, so it has to. It isn't so much the content of your life experiences that becomes revealed – as it would be in therapy – but your modus operandi towards life: how you go about things, how you deal with success and failure, what makes you anxious and fearful, how you deal with a challenge.

I couldn't count the number of teachers whose work I have personally experienced. Some of them helped me to create a sense of being more myself, while others left me feeling how they looked. Some of them had almost no effect, while still others induced deep emotions not normally accessible to me.

How a teacher affects you is dependent upon three factors:

1. their skill as a teacher

2. your receptivity as a student

3. the chemistry of both of your personalities.

The teacher's skill

Chapter 5 explores the different styles of teaching you can encounter which suit different personalities, but the all-important question is: did you learn anything?

Alexander work is an educational process so it's not asking too much that you learn something, even in your first lesson. Some teachers will insist that Alexander work is too complicated, too experientially based, and it is naive to think anyone can learn anything in just one lesson. I don't agree with that – I take the radical position, thanks to my teacher Marj, that the Alexander work is simple. It's our old habits that are complicated!

However, your learning may not be intellectual – it could be ontological. Alexander hands-on work affects your being, your sense of self. As one teacher puts it, you cease being who you imagine yourself to be and become who you are. It's a paradigm shift that defies our everyday conception of learning.

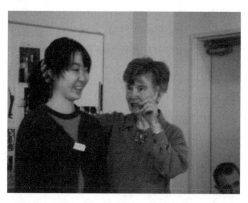

Elisabeth Walker, shown here teaching in Japan in 2002, was then one of only a handful of teachers left in the world who were trained by Alexander before his death in 1955. Photo by Akihiro Tada.

Of course, not every lesson will be as profound as that. You may just learn a simple thing – such as how you pull your head back all the time and that's why your neck gets stiff. In some ways, that can be of more practical value than the 'big experience'. Either way, your teacher should be able to get something across to you and not leave you completely mystified, although Alexander work is always a little mysterious, if only because we are human.

Your receptivity as a student

This is more important than you think it is, because the success of Alexander work is in direct ratio to your own receptivity to it. A good Alexander teacher actually doesn't 'do' anything to you – although it sure looks and feels as if they do. As I will explain further on, a teacher is inducing your nervous system to behave in a particular way. For that to succeed, you need to cooperate. If you're cynical, looking for fault and wanting to gain evidence for a negative outcome, you will probably find it.

Alexander work is so subtle that some people at first think nothing's happening and it must be one great big sham. Certainly, as a young teacher, I was afraid my pupils would think that! One friend who trained told me that he didn't feel much during his first year of lessons, so there's a small chance that this will happen to you. However, if your mind is closed, it is unlikely you will ever feel much happening and will come to think that all this talk of 'new experiences' and 'giving directions' is just so much psycho-babble. My friend persisted because he believed there was something to get and, being a dancer, he was determined to get it. Motivation is everything.

I have also had the misfortune to work with pupils who came not at their bidding but because an insurance company or office manager insisted they take lessons. Not a good idea – these pupils were the toughest I've ever had because they simply didn't want to be there. You'd think, because many of them were in great pain, that they'd be desperate for any help they could get.

At least, that's what I naively thought when I took on such a project many years ago. There was a great lesson there for me and now I make a point of helping my pupils sort out exactly what they want from their lessons. It differs a lot and it affects the way I teach them, so it is important. I strongly suggest you think through that simple, little step before you approach a teacher and that you communicate it to them the first time you meet.

The chemistry of your personalities

Some people want to be told; others definitely don't. Some pupils want to please their teachers; others couldn't care less. We are all so different and the pedagogy of Alexander teachers reflects this: there are all kinds of teachers and teaching styles.

If you're someone who just likes to absorb what's going on and listen, then don't stick with a teacher who prods you all the time, especially if it creates anxiety on your part. If you feel anxiety during a lesson, you are in no state to learn anything. Once I taught in a much more confrontational style, demanding that my students take responsibility for themselves by challenging them to tell me what they thought was going on. Later I realized that exciting a pupil's fear reflexes wasn't really a smart way of helping them to take responsibility for themselves, so I softened my approach and practised a little more patience.

Is your teacher patient with you? It's important to feel you have the space and time to make mistakes. Otherwise, you will enter a trying-to-please mode of behaviour and that's fatal to Alexander lessons. In Alexander lessons you are learning to change the habits of a lifetime and to do that it's important to have a sense of support. Support, however, can appear in many different ways depending on your personal outlook.

For example, I like a teacher who calls a spade a spade – my teacher Marj was like that. She'd even smack me if I got out of line! In a playful way, but sometimes in dead earnest – I'd get scolded and smacked. Now, a lot of people couldn't contend with that – even ideologically, if not emotionally.

They thought such behaviour on the part of Marj was wrong. But I didn't react that way. First, I realized Marj was born in 1899 and grew up with very different values from my own. Second, and more to the point, I knew that Marj's actions were entirely motivated by a desire to help me learn – and I wanted to learn. There was no anger behind her smacks – only compassion. So, no problem. It didn't hurt and actually I thought it was quite funny. We'd laugh about it together.

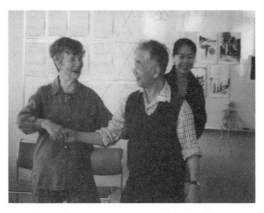

Here Elisabeth is having fun while working with translator Yuzuru Katagiri. In Alexander lessons you need to feel you have the time and space to make mistakes, and enjoy doing it! Photo by Akihiro Tada.

Alexander was known to have literally thrown people out of his teaching room because they wouldn't pay attention to their lessons. I've not heard of that happening these days – teachers could get sued – but I would have enjoyed a challenge like that. Maybe you wouldn't; maybe I'm warped – who knows? This isn't about judgements; it's about what works for you right now.

Alexander teachers are human beings and can be as insecure as the next person, so make sure the chemistry with your teacher works for you. If it does, your experiences will deepen with each lesson. If not, you will always be protecting a little bit of yourself, and 'protection' is nothing else but a kind of tension. Alexander lessons aren't like anything else so it's important to get the right teacher before you settle into regular lessons.

Your teacher's hands-on work

Your teacher will touch you. Continuously. How will you feel about that?

Here is a story that illustrates how special this touch is. Over the years I have conducted many experiments putting my Alexander hands-on skills to work with horses. Actually, most of them love it – I've had them nuzzle me with their heads to get me to continue doing my hands-on work with them. It's a heart-warming experience. However, I did observe one curious resistance: they did not like me to touch them with Alexander hands at the place of an injury. The strange thing about this is that I could stroke them or pat them in a normal kind of way at the same spot, but as soon as I put my hands on with Alexander intentions they pulled away. It was as if they instinctively knew that those Alexander hands could mess around with their insides in a way that a normal stroking or patting never could.

Alexander hands-on work does mess around with your insides – it calibrates the automated programs of coordination and, with a skilful teacher, you can it feel happen despite yourself. The more skilful the teacher, the less you have to think yourself. There's a story of Alexander, in his later years, walking out from a lesson, looking at his hands and remarking something along the lines that he didn't need his pupils to think any more because his hands could do everything for them.

I regularly train Alexander teachers and have done for years. One of their first lessons when they are starting to put hands on is to distinguish three ways in which they can use their hands on pupils:

1. to listen

2. to invite

3. to tell.

It will be useful to analyze these in turn. As a pupil, it is going to help if you understand what your teacher is setting out to do with their hands. It is unique.

Listening hands

Every teacher must train to do this. It is difficult to explain if you've never had a lesson, but the best metaphor I can think of is this. Imagine you are using your hands to maintain an object in balance through its own axis as shown in Figure 5.1. You don't want to support any of its weight – nor can you lean on it, as it would fall the other way. So both you and the object maintain an independent balance.

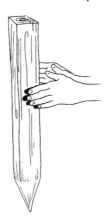

Figure 5.1 Listening hands – as the object sways you can maintain it in balance by sensing and counteracting it before it falls too far without having to bear its weight.

At the same time as there is this independence between you and the object, there is paradoxically an *interdependence* of balance occurring. For example, every time the object begins to fall off its balance, you gently correct it. Every time you feel that you are leaning too much and it begins to fall the other way, you must correct that too. It is only by listening to the balance of the object that you are able to make these continuous corrections. The sooner you sense the change and counteract it, the less effort is required on your part.

Alexander teachers are trained to listen to your coordination in that way. They can pick up an incredible amount of information about the continuously occurring shifts of balance in your coordination and, with that information, move to utilize the second aspect of their skill.

Inviting hands

When you reach Chapter 7, you will become familiar with the wide variety of directions that different parts of your body can be moving in while you are standing. Standing is an activity, a process of adjustment and readjustment. Sir Charles Sherrington, a Nobel laureate and early 20th-century physiologist who made favourable remarks about Alexander's work, once pointed out that the human being in the act of standing is constantly at the edge of catastrophe. Watching the first steps of an emerging toddler is testament to that. It's what one contemporary American dancer calls 'the inner dance'.

So the Alexander teacher's hands are listening to that inner dance you are making all the time: your head falling back, your neck pushing down, your rib cage collapsing and arching at the lower back, your hips thrusting forward, knees locking. I haven't even begun to describe all the various subtle variations that are contained within each of these larger movements.

Having understood the pattern of coordination you are currently making, the teacher then uses his or her hands to talk to your nervous system directly and invite it to make a different kind of inner dance, one that doesn't cause so much downward pressure and tension in your body. This can be quite a complex invitation, because every second millions upon millions of motor neurons are causing excitation in millions upon millions of muscle fibres in response to millions upon millions of continuously changing conditions. It's a surprise that an Alexander teacher's hands can get a word in at all! It takes three years of training for an Alexander teacher to have even this basic skill in their hands. It takes a lifetime to perfect.

Why doesn't a teacher ask you out straight out to coordinate yourself in the way their hands are inviting you to? Wouldn't that be quicker than fussing around with all this hands-on work? Actually, a good teacher will – but only after they have used their hands to induce in you the sensation of coordination they want you to experience. The reason for this is simple: 'you' aren't the one coordinating yourself. I mean, think about it: do you really control, or even sense, all these subtle shifts and changes that are occurring every second in your head, neck, chest, pelvis, arms, legs and jaw while you are reading this book? Can you feel all that happening right now? Of course not. We have no idea what's going on. In fact, as Alexander put it, 'we do not know how we use ourselves any more than the dog or cat knows'.

Something is guiding this inner dance and if it isn't 'you', then who is it? Well, of course it's you but not the conscious, volitional aspect of yourself that most of us identify with. This inner dance is being controlled by brain centres below the conscious or cortical level – what some people might call the sub-conscious self – in centres with scary names like the basal ganglia, mesencephalon and metencephalon. Luckily, these centres are open to suggestion, so the Alexander teacher's hands are inviting them to dance together in an integrated way. If things go well, and you cooperate with this invitation, you soon feel a change in your body. This is the sensation that your Alexander teacher is inviting you to experience.

Telling hands

If the teacher's hands can't engage your mind, you'll never move. That's where your cooperation is so essential. There are few teachers in the world who possess the skill that Alexander was renowned to have had in his hands. He could take you out of a chair by placing one hand on the top of your head and then literally draw you up into standing by the sheer force of the direction in his hands. It felt (I was told) that he was miraculously sucking you up out of the chair despite yourself.

I've yet to experience such a thing myself, but when a teacher's hands are really effective, they do tell your coordination what to do. You watch the results in amazement as your body transforms without you seeming to do anything. It really is quite the most remarkable thing to feel and it's why people get addicted to their lessons. It just feels so good.

But telling hands can become pushy hands and this is something I warn all my trainee teachers to watch. It isn't nearly so pleasant an experience to have a teacher manipulate you into a pattern of coordination that he or she feels is the right one for you. You can go away from the lesson feeling like your teacher looks and it just isn't you. This can happen if the teacher is impatient, or a little bossy, or just too full of his or her own ideas about what is right and wrong. You have to be the judge of that. Lessons need to be giving you tangible benefits, so if they are, continue on.

The crux of the matter is that a good teacher doesn't know what is right for you – that's too presumptuous and, sadly, there are too many practitioners of all kinds who think that they do know. What we, as Alexander teachers, know is what isn't beneficial for you. Alexander remarked:

'To know when we are wrong is all that we shall ever know in this world.'

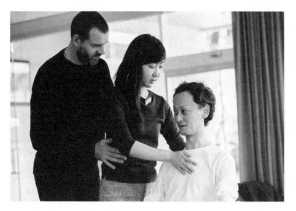

In his training school in Japan, Jeremy is shown here leading students through the four-year process of learning to coordinate their touch for teaching the Alexander Technique. Photo by Akihiro Tada.

It's learning how to stop the wrong thing from happening that emancipates the right direction into action. To achieve this, a teacher's hands talk directly to your locomotive system, while our words appeal to your conscious mind, so that together both pupil and teacher can learn how to prevent the mosaic of inappropriate movements that have collectively resulted in the condition of mal-coordination that brought you to the lesson in the first place. 'All you'll get', my teacher Marj used to remind us, 'is the absence of what you had.' And then there'd be a little twinkle in her eye.

The actual lesson

Depending upon the lineage of your teacher, a lesson can proceed in many different ways. I will discuss these differences at length in Chapter 5. Here I will describe the central components of any Alexander lesson, regardless of the style your teacher is working in. Maybe some of these components will be missing from your lesson – well, ask yourself the question: am I learning? If the answer is yes, keep it up. Every teacher has a right to develop his or her own methodology and it may not be exactly as I have described here. Thank goodness for variety. This is how I give a lesson.

Every lesson has one purpose of offering you a new sensation. This is a sensation of coordinating yourself in an initially unfamiliar but easier and more natural manner. A good teacher will give you a taste of this experience in your first lesson. However, if that was all the lesson was about, we wouldn't be calling ourselves teachers.

More importantly, each lesson seeks to put that new sensation into a context that you can understand. You are there to learn how to generate this sensation for yourself. These two elements are achieved through a delicate interplay between three processes:

1. observation

2. interpretation

3. experimentation.

These three processes are in turn applied to three different kinds of activities, known in Alexander jargon as:

1. chairwork

2. tablework

3. activities.

I'll give a brief description of these three activities, and then investigate how observation, interpretation and experimentation are related to them to achieve the two outcomes of a lesson.

Chairwork

This is the classic activity around which most Alexander teachers centre their lessons. It involves you getting in and out of a chair with the teacher's assistance and each time gives rise to a new result. I once had an eccentric, older man with a big, bushy moustache come for a lesson and at its finish, as he was exiting the door, he stopped suddenly, turned back, looked at the chair, at me, shook his head and declared, 'What an extraordinary way to earn a living!'

It is extraordinary. Where else would you pay a lot of money to learn how to get out of a chair? About this Alexander remarked:

> 'It's not getting in and out of chairs even under the best of conditions that is of any value; that is simply physical culture – it is what you have been doing in preparation that counts when it comes to making movements.'

So, actually, you aren't learning how to get out of a chair – this is a device, a method, not an end in itself. You are learning how to inhibit an inappropriate reaction to a stimulus (in this case to sit or to stand) in order to bring about a condition of coordination that is more beneficial. Once you have learnt this procedure, you can apply it anywhere, anytime, to anything. Alexander said:

> 'If you apply the principle to the carrying out of one evolution, you have learned the lot.'

Tablework

Pupils love tablework. You lie down on your back in semi-supine position – with your knees bent up and your head resting on some books – while the teacher gently helps to lengthen your torso, arms and legs. A longer description of this appears in Chapter 6, under the heading 'Semi-supine procedure'. Also see Figure 6.4.

Some teachers will work on you silently; others will chat away about everything. Some will give you guided instructions as to what to think and still others will ask you to actively participate in different procedures and activities – all as you remain lying on your back in semi-supine.

Alexander did very little tablework, although he didn't disapprove of or discourage it. He is reported to have remarked to teachers that if you can't get what you want with the pupil in upright, then put them on the table and work. Alexander was so good he didn't need to do tablework – I imagine he could get more changes with his hands in one minute than I can in 30! Despite our namesake, we're not all multiple Alexanders, so tablework has become an essential tool of an Alexander lesson.

My personal view of tablework is that sometimes pupils become too attached to it. It is more therapeutic than educational and, while there's nothing wrong with that, Alexander lessons are supposed to be teaching you something, not just making you feel good. I have heard of teachers doing nothing else but tablework and that surprises me. I am not sure how you learn to coordinate yourself differently from lessons that consist of you lying passively on your back the entire time. I know that some teachers argue that you can. Alexander himself used to get tough with pupils who spent too much time in semi-supine. He'd send his assistants to get them up with the comment 'They are only lazing there.' Enjoy tablework, but realize it is less of a substitute and more of a support to the real work of your lessons.

Semi-supine, however, is probably the closest you'll ever get to having a definite routine that you can practise. This is another puzzling thing about your lessons: while there are many different activities you can explore, there are no set exercises that you can go home and show others or practise on your own.

Explain to someone what happened in your lesson and their eyes will eventually glaze over. A lesson is about changing the state of your consciousness and, as such, is best understood through experience alone. Lessons teach you how to keep applying the three processes – observation, interpretation and experimentation – in order to gain this experience, regardless of the type of activity you are doing.

Activities

Chairwork is an activity, but, aside from that, most teachers will at least explore walking, bending and doing things with your arms. However, a large portion of Alexander teachers don't explore much more than that, but, then, neither did Alexander. Remember, it is the principles being used to change your coordination, not the activity itself, that is the focus of learning. Ultimately, it doesn't matter what activity you do.

That said, it is often of value to explore Alexander's discoveries in relation to specialized activities such as playing a musical instrument, dancing, making pots or especially to any activity you are involved in regularly as part of your daily life. It is of value because if you examine this in your Alexander lesson, the activity itself will serve as a reminder to apply what you are learning. I once saw my teacher Marj help a woman put some overalls on! Ask your Alexander teacher if you can do some activities with them. While some may not be accustomed to teaching in this way, most will be willing to explore this with you. See 'The teaching style' headings in Chapter 5 for more information on this point.

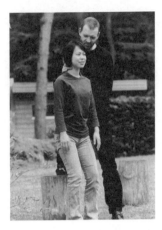

Chairwork: The author works with a student on the movement of sitting. In Alexander lessons you are guided in everyday movements and study how to redirect your energy. Photo by Akihiro Tada.

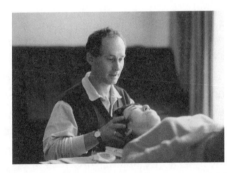

Tablework: On a trip to Japan, Peter Grunwald leads a student through his Vision and Eyesight application of the Alexander Technique. Photo by Akihiro Tada.

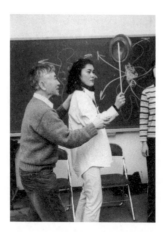

Activities: Here Yuzuru Katagiri has found an exciting way to explore the concept of balance with his student. Learning through activities can open the lesson up to originality and fun. Photo by Akihiro Tada.

Observation

My teacher Marj once told me: 'I don't teach my pupils anything until they have made an observation for themselves.' So, at the start of the lesson, you will be asked to offer any observations you have about your coordination as you get in and out of the chair. This may be done before the teacher works on you or after the teacher works on you. You may initially be perplexed by this request – what, you wonder, am I supposed to observe?

Pupils often say things like 'I pushed up out of the chair' or 'It felt hard.' Of course, these aren't observations; they're interpretations. The first aspect of your learning is to appreciate the difference between an observation and an interpretation. If you say something like 'I pushed up' – pushed what? Be specific. Your arms? Your legs? If you say something like 'It was hard', that isn't an observation; that's a subjective judgement based upon your experience.

What was the actual experience you had – can you describe that? What were the elements that lead you to interpret it as 'hard'? When we come to understand these elements, it becomes possible to alter them, or at least experiment with altering them.

Here's a rough definition of observation that I use for my pupils. I ask them to imagine they are explaining what they did to a blind person. Words like 'hard' and 'pushy' are difficult to imagine accurately – they could mean anything – but if you said something like 'I pulled my knees together and lifted my shoulders as I pressed down with my hands on to my upper legs', then our blind friend would be closer to understanding what you actually did, as opposed to how you felt about it.

My teacher Marj taught that one aspect of an Alexander lesson is to learn a new language. You develop a vocabulary with which you can confidently navigate the terrain of your coordination. A surgeon friend of mine once declared that a London cab driver knew as much as he did: they both knew the name, location and connections of hundreds of objects and used this knowledge to help others. The principle was the same, he claimed – it was only the vocabulary, their objects and what was at stake that differed. In that way, Alexander lessons slowly define a new vocabulary; in this case, the objects are sensations and movements.

The process of observation is about giving names to all these new sensations – discerning categories and creating descriptions which didn't exist previously. Slowly, based on our observations, we build up a vocabulary to better understand, and communicate about, our coordination.

However, observations of themselves are not much use. They need to be understood within a wider context. A time comes when it is necessary to consider these observations and ask: how we can interpret them?

Interpretation

'This chair is uncomfortable.' How often have you heard that said? People everywhere, every day, make statements like that. Maybe you have too at one time. Yet behind this view is an interpretation that is unhelpful, for it deprives you of direct control by making the chair more powerful than you. However, I didn't say it wasn't true – it's an interpretation, so it's as true as you want it to be.

What's an alternative interpretation? How about 'I do something to myself when I sit in this particular chair that causes me to feel discomfort'? Now who's responsible? Not the chair. You just took responsibility for yourself and stopped blaming that inanimate thing. While this responsibility may not be as comforting to live with, it does offer you a line of escape; within that interpretation, a different kind of action is available to you.

Now, instead of spending your energy looking for the perfect chair, you can occupy yourself more usefully by discovering what you do to cause your discomfort and learn to stop it. Think of it this way: does every person have exactly the same experience of discomfort that you do when they sit in that chair? Of course not. So that suggests that your discomfort doesn't really come from the chair's side alone, even though that's how it might feel to you. It also comes from your side, from something *you are doing* in reaction to the chair. Your Alexander teacher will help you discover what – it is one reason to take lessons in the first place. The way that you discover that something is by experimenting with different sensations of sitting in that chair, guided by your Alexander teacher's hands.

Experimentation

The proof of the pudding is in the eating. Personally, I love to take a pupil who is thinking, 'This chair is uncomfortable' and work on them till they do feel comfortable. Then I ask, 'Oh, by the way, is the chair still making you feel uncomfortable?' Now that it isn't, the pupil can realize the shortcomings of their previous way of thinking and start taking responsibility for more of their experiences.

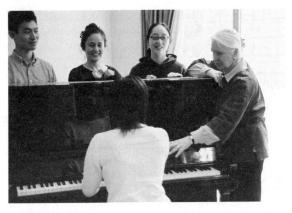

Experimenting: Vivien Mackie, an Alexander teacher and accomplished cellist from London, shown here helping a Japanese musician experiment with Alexander principles. Photo by Akihiro Tada.

This particular procedure is an example of an experiment designed to change a pupil's interpretation or thinking. A good Alexander lesson should be full of such experiments: where your old idea is challenged by a new experience, causing you to rethink your habitual reaction by making a decision to respond to it differently in the future. Alexander said:

> 'Boiled down, it all comes to inhibiting a particular reaction to a given stimulus. But no one will see it that way. They will all see it as getting in and out of a chair the right way. It is nothing of the kind. It is that a pupil decided what he will or will not consent to do.'

In your lesson you will come to understand how to apply the concepts of direction, inhibition and faulty sensory perception in your everyday life. Although I analyzed these three concepts while relating Alexander's story in Chapter 2, I will briefly mention them here in the context of an Alexander lesson.

Direction

This word can have a number of different meanings, even in the context of Alexander's discoveries. In a lesson, it refers mainly to the four directions that are explained at length in Chapters 3 and 7 – the *how* of thinking as well as the *what* you are thinking about. Alexander teachers also talk a lot about 'doing' and 'non-doing' with regard to giving directions. These are subtle shades of meaning on this word 'direction'. Didn't I warn you there's a whole new vocabulary to learn?

Doing directions are the kind everyone does when they are trying to 'sit up straight', 'pull the shoulders back', 'chin up' – all that sort of thing. They can be defined as thoughts that result in deliberately tightened muscles.

Non-doing directions are inhibitory in nature: they aim to prevent certain patterns of contraction; thus they can be defined as thoughts that result in the inhibition of unnecessary contractions.

Inhibition

Notice I used that word in the last sentence: 'the inhibition of unnecessary contractions'. Just as with the word 'direction', 'inhibition' has many meanings, even in an Alexander context. In the sense of inhibiting muscles, it is necessary to understand that this is a positive biological function of certain motor neurons. It is not to be equated with suppression which is quite a different thing. I will briefly recap some of the information in Chapter 3.

Excitation and inhibition are two technical names that physiologists use to describe the function of a motor neuron – one of the essential components of our locomotive system. Prior to the discovery of inhibition, physiologists used to think that motor neurons only excited muscles to contract. It was quite revolutionary to discover that there were actually motor neurons devoted to the inhibition of muscle contraction.

Alexander discovered this empirically long before the physiologists proved it in the laboratory. He quickly realized that if he could inhibit one set of reactions, it released a new coordination into being. To do it any other way simply meant he would merely be layering one set of contractions on top of an older uninhibited set. Alexander said:

'You can't do what you don't know if you keep doing what you do know.'

So, in Alexander lessons, *first* you discover what are the habitual directions you are giving to yourself, *then* you learn to inhibit those directions and *instead* give the new Alexander directions in the way your Alexander teacher's hands are guiding you.

There also is a profound meaning to inhibition, beyond this physiology, although this is still the basis of any change we make. Changing a simple habit of coordination might involve us in letting go of an identity that we have built up of ourselves – all the emotional complexities inherent in achieving this. I explore this in greater depth in Chapter 3, under the heading 'Emotional patterns of coordination', but essentially it means that this identity is in fact a false view of ourselves, a view that is based on our sensory appreciation, and it may be the cause of the trouble that first brought us to lessons. Alexander said:

> 'Sensory appreciation conditions conception – you can't know a thing by an instrument that is wrong.'

Faulty sensory appreciation

It is extremely important to understand this concept of Alexander's. The key aspect of this concept is that it says your appreciation or interpretation of the event is faulty. It doesn't mean your perception of the actual event is faulty. It's an example of where our observations and our interpretations of them have collapsed themselves together so they appear to our mind as the same thing, when in fact they are different.

The concept is best understood initially in psychological terms that we are all familiar with. If Beatrice tells Tony, Ingrid and Sally to be quiet, that is an event. None of those four will dispute that Beatrice said that. As far as hearing or seeing, there's nothing faulty about their senses. However, how does each interpret that event? Well, Tony thinks that Beatrice is being bossy and has it in for him. Sally, on the other hand, is happy, because she perceives that Beatrice is trying to help them all. Ingrid is puzzled – she's just met them all and wonders just why Beatrice is saying that. One event, three different perceptions. Who's right?

That's where we leave this example, for the criteria to determine who's right becomes complex, even impossible to define. Luckily, as far as our coordination goes, it is easy to define what is right. What is right is what leads us towards freedom, flexibility and general good health.

However, many ideas of what is right are at odds with this. An example is that many people feel that a slump is relaxed. Relaxed? A slump? When did slumping for two hours ever leave you feeling relaxed? Think about it. We get stiff, tired and sore from slumping. It is an odd idea to think that slumping is relaxing.

Yet that is our appreciation of it; that is how we think about it when we slump and, in Alexander's terms, that appreciation or thinking is faulty. To us, we feel as if we are relaxing when we slump, yet all the objective evidence refutes that. Still, even knowing this, we still feel that way. We need to re-educate this feeling or belief. We need Alexander lessons.

There's a story of Alexander working on a young girl who was quite physically distorted in her movements but, after being straightened up in a lesson with Alexander, she ran over to her mother, crying, 'Mummy, Mummy, the man's made me all crooked!' Of course she felt crooked because her idea of straight was crooked. Alexander was literally setting her straight by giving an experience to her of what straight is. Alexander once put it more bluntly:

'All the dammed fools in the world believe they are actually doing what they think they are doing.'

This phenomenon of faulty sensory appreciation is the greatest obstacle to anyone attempting to work by themselves without a teacher's assistance. In Alexander terms, your idea of right is the very thing that needs to change. Yet it's all you have to guide you to change. To make a successful change, you need first to experience the wrongness of your right. Difficult to do on your own. Alexander said:

'Everyone wants to be right, but no one stops to consider if their idea of right is right.'

How many lessons?

Whenever anyone asks me this question these days, I ask them: how many lessons does it take to learn the piano?

Learning the piano is no more complicated than learning how to coordinate your body, so the question becomes: what do you want to gain? Do you want to be a concert pianist (Alexander teacher) or do you just want to play a ten-finger exercise (help yourself)? If you have sustained a recent injury, then even one lesson can be of tremendous help. If you have had a chronic problem all your life, then you may need to be taking occasional lessons for the rest of your life. Most pupils fall between those two extremes. In the end, it depends on your motivation, your aim and your application, just like learning the piano.

But it is interesting to look at Alexander himself. What did he ask of his pupils? A friend of mine once took lessons from him in the early 1950s, not long before his death in 1955. At that time, this is his recollection of Alexander's terms. First: read all his books. (My friend didn't and Alexander never asked.) Second: a minimum of 30 lessons. Third: for the first 20 lessons, take five lessons per week, Monday to Friday, 30 minutes each; for the final ten lessons, two lessons a week. Fourth: pay in advance.

I know of no teacher who dictates terms like that these days but, then, no one is Alexander either. However, the 30 lessons is still conventional wisdom, although few teachers these days will insist upon it before accepting you as a pupil. However, when you consider that an Alexander teacher spends the equivalent of 3,200 private lessons to gain a qualification to teach, 30 lessons is nothing at all.

How much?

About the same as dinner and a movie, wherever you live. Alexander lessons aren't cheap, but neither is a visit to the therapist. Of course, Alexander lessons are on-going for quite a while so they represent an investment in yourself. A full series of lessons equals the cost of buying yourself a luxury item or going on a holiday. However, lessons are likely to give you far more joy and enduring value for your money.

If you commit for a lot of lessons in advance, some teachers will give you a discount. If they don't offer, ask. No harm in that.

Where?

These days you will often find an Alexander teacher working in a centre with a variety of other therapists. I used to teach in a place like this – we had a doctor, three psychologists, a nutritionist, two chiropractors and me. Less commonly, there are some exclusively Alexander centres where you can get lessons or go to groups. Alexander centres are usually places where a teacher training school operates, and if that's the case, it's often possible to get cheap, even free lessons, with final-year students.

However, the vast majority of Alexander teachers work out of their homes. This may seem odd at first, especially for a person charging professional fees, but, unlike other professionals in the medical and para-medical field, Alexander teachers don't consider themselves therapists. We're more in the nature of music teachers and a lot of them work out of their homes too.

However, as they do get healing results, Alexander teachers exist in a kind of medical limbo. While they insist they are teachers, many of their pupils see them as therapists who are helping them to get better. It's a constant dilemma for Alexander teachers, for, despite their own self-image, they do manage to get mixed up with medical insurance and the like. Perhaps coming to their home helps underline the fact that you are their pupil, not their patient.

When you enter their teaching room, there will most probably be three things: a chair, a table and a mirror. The chair is for chairwork, the table for tablework and the mirror is for you to see that, as the lesson progresses, you don't actually look at all like the way you feel you must be looking.

The teacher will touch you but with your clothes on – if he or she wants you to take them off, get out of there pretty quick. It isn't necessary and it is not done. Also, teachers do not need to touch your genitals, breasts or bottom – report the teacher if he or she tries things like that with you.

Conclusion

When you start lessons, make sure you wait until you are sure that you can follow them through for a while. The effect of lessons tends to build exponentially, week by week, but if you keep cancelling lessons and putting them off, you can lose that effect. Every lesson becomes about dragging you back to the standard you reached at the end of the previous one. Some Alexander teachers will even refuse to teach you unless you begin twice a week. This depends on both the teacher and your reason for taking lessons.

It is a good idea to keep a journal. Progress can seem slow until you look back and realize how much has changed. In Alexander lessons, you are always intrigued by the next problem, so it is sometimes too easy to forget just how far along you have actually progressed. A journal will help to keep your perspective on the process.

Finally, Alexander lessons can be great fun – and a real adventure. They will open you up to an entire new domain of knowledge about yourself, a new universe of experience that beckons to be understood. As this world reveals itself to you, there can be amazing and unexpected results. Almost everyone is impressed by their Alexander lessons and become their best ambassador. Alexander was a genius and has bestowed on us a marvellous legacy. Don't miss out.

Teaching Lineages

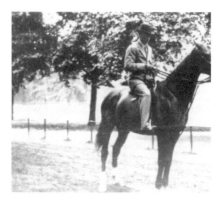

Alexander was an enthusiastic horse rider and his
technique is used today as part of the training of
equestrian riders on the German Olympic team.

'Don't come to me unless, when I tell you you
are wrong, you make up your mind to smile and
be pleased.'

F. M. Alexander

The Alexander work evolves more like a martial art than a
remedial art. Its development more closely resembles that of
aikido than chiropractic. Although there is no formal ranking
system, still there are a number of terms used by teachers to
denote a particular status. At the top you have the 'master
teachers', who may loosely be defined as the founders of
the primary teaching lineages that currently exist in the
Alexander world. Then you have 'senior teachers', 'directors

of training schools', 'sponsoring teachers', 'junior teachers', 'second-generation teachers' and many other descriptive terms along those lines – not unlike the various coloured 'belts' found in the martial arts.

The Alexander world's version of a 'black belt' is becoming a Director of a training school. Directors are an influential group and meet and discuss issues regularly in many countries. To qualify, you must have been teaching between seven and ten years, depending on the rules of the individual society, and be recognized as a person with the necessary skills to both teach and organize a teacher training school.

No one comes out of high school and trains to be an Alexander teacher as a career. The training is a considerable investment, both in time and money, so most teachers are highly motivated to understand and apply this work to themselves. For most teachers, it's a decision of personal growth and development. Quite a few trainees continue with their original occupation upon qualification – as a dancer, singer, yoga teacher, musician or suchlike – using their new skills to help others in their chosen field. Occasionally, they don't teach at all – instead concentrating on applying what they have learnt to enhance their own skill.

Your teacher's qualifications

There are two independent networks that oversee teacher registration, training and general standards. The largest is the international network of Alexander Technique Affiliated Societies – affiliated because, while they all recognize each other's members, each still exists as a separate organization with its own constitution, by-laws and standards. The second network is one organization that calls itself Alexander Technique International (ATI) and, as the name suggests, it consists of members spread across the world. Some teachers belong to both groups. ATI differs from the Affiliated Societies because it operates under a radically different set of ground rules for the training of teachers.

The Affiliated Societies currently exist in America, Australia, Belgium, Canada, Denmark, France, Germany, Israel, Netherlands, South Africa, Switzerland and the UK – see the Resources at the end of the book. They have what is called 'the 1,600 hour standard'. This means that any teacher on a training course approved by one of these Societies must have completed 1,600 hours of training under quite strict conditions. These conditions include teacher-to-trainee ratios, ratio of practical teaching to theoretical study, prerequisites to be a Director of Training and a host of other by-laws, guidelines and constitutional imperatives.

ATI takes a radically different approach. It got out of the business of regulating training schools altogether and instead has 'Sponsoring Members' who are recognized by their peers as outstanding teachers with experience in teacher training. To become a Sponsoring Member of ATI, you must submit at an AGM of the full Teaching Membership the guidelines and criteria you will use to assess applicants for Teaching Membership. If your proposal receives a majority vote, then you become a Sponsoring Teacher Member of ATI.

Three of these Sponsoring Members must recommend a trainee for membership before ATI will register them as a Teaching Member. In practice, ATI training schools also run over three years and have adopted the '1,600 standard'. However, they offer more part-time courses over longer periods and differ in other subtle ways. In practice, a 'Sponsoring Member' is ATI's equivalent of the Affiliated Society's 'Director of Training'.

Of course, there's politics involved here – when isn't there? ATI tends to be the more 'liberal' wing of the Alexander community; the Affiliated Societies more 'conservative'. ATI has a lot of teachers who rejected the status quo and wanted to explore alternatives together. For example, the Affiliated Societies at present won't countenance part-time training, whereas there are several schools structured this way under the ATI umbrella. Also, the unconventional 'apprenticeship' training methods of Marjorie Barstow did not conform to the Affiliated Societies rule books, so many of her teachers participated in setting up ATI and are now members of it.

Although it's possible to find poor practitioners in either group, I do not think the differences should be of any concern to you when looking for a teacher. A member of either meets a professional standard and will be as competent as their own skills allow them to be. Base your assessment on the rapport you can make with your teacher, their skill, together with convenience and price. See Chapter 4 for a detailed discussion on how to choose a teacher.

The teaching lineages

Since his death, Alexander's work has spawned a number of teaching lineages which are identified by their namesakes. Each of these lineages has a distinctive style – often in keeping with the founder's own personality – and in this chapter I will briefly introduce you to three major lineages.

I might add that this is a risky thing for me to do because each lineage, of course, feels that it is the only one that is true to the originator and is not a 'lineage' at all. I can expect some bad press for attempting this in a few Alexander journals and maybe even the odd cross letter. I've made clear my own 'lineage' lest the reader suspects I am being sly. I will try to be fair but I cannot say with complete confidence that I am qualified to be making these judgements, but then I am not sure anyone else is either. My only real qualification for this task is that I have personally supervised a special issue of *direction*, the journal that I published, on each of these Master teachers and, in the course of editing each edition, have had many discussions and experiences with teachers from all three lineages.

So what the heck – I think you will find it interesting and useful to know a little of the history of the Alexander work. Like any other profession, it has its politics.

As far as the 'politics' of it goes, the further the link back to the Master teacher, the more reluctant a teacher will be to acknowledge the line of their teaching. If you ask them, it is just as likely that they will dismiss your question as irrelevant – or at least be put out by it. This is understandable: people don't like to be categorized. Everyone is an individual and these days there has been far more 'cross-breeding' than in the past. Teachers will resist being pigeonholed by you – particularly when they hear you read it in a book!

An example of this is that the Society of Teachers of the Alexander Technique in England – the world's largest Society of Teachers – used to list teachers with a code indicating who they had trained with. They received a flood of complaints from Teaching Members about this practice and it was dropped.

Although the lineages all still exist in their purest forms, there is also a lot of grey. Also, there is now a whole new generation of teachers putting their own stamp on the work that I make no mention of. These are tomorrow's 'Masters' and they may feel they have their own unique brand of Alexander work. So exercise caution with this information – it is merely a background guide, not a definitive plan.

Walter Carrington (1915–2005)

A brief biography

Walter Carrington continued to live and run a teacher training school in London until a few weeks before his death in 2005. Of the three lineages I am reviewing, he was the last of the Master teachers to pass on. His contribution to the development of the work has been enormous.

Born the son of a clergyman in Yorkshire in 1915, Mr Carrington originally planned to join the Order of the Jesuits. Although his life took a different path, he still exuded a quiet serenity and had the happy knack of not making enemies. Although I never knew Alexander – he died before I was born – I do know that his life is littered with stories of irreconcilable breaks between him and his once-trusted lieutenants. But not Mr Carrington: he managed to maintain a trusting and close relationship with Alexander right through to the end, and then carried on the training school after Alexander's death.

It was his form master at St Paul's who first introduced Mr Carrington to Alexander's work, but it was the successful lessons of his mother – who suffered from chronic indigestion and was returned to health by a course of lessons with Alexander – that convinced him that this was a worthy vocation. He qualified in 1939 and immediately began assisting Alexander on the training course while developing a private practice of individual lessons.

During the war he flew with the RAF until his plane was shot down over Hungary and he was taken prisoner. He suffered horrific injuries, including a fractured pelvis and collar bone, and was transferred to a military hospital, eventually to make his way home. In his later years, you could notice that he still suffered from the effects of these war injuries – what was remarkable was that he remained upright at all!

After the war finished, he pretty much stayed with Alexander, holding the fort while Alexander made his many trips to America. Mr Carrington became the rock that held Alexander's training school together.

Mr Carrington was also the only one of the Master teachers to be around Alexander during a significant development in Alexander's 'hands-on work'. At the age of 79, Alexander suffered a stroke and for the next 12 months worked to restore the use of one side of his body. His paralysis and general weakness meant he had no more physical strength to use. In response to this, he developed a powerful hands-on touch which relied less on physical support and more on the focus and clarity of his direction – as discussed in Chapter 4, 'An Alexander Lesson'.

This exceptionally light yet powerful non-doing touch is a feature of many Carrington teachers. It certainly influenced me as I began my training in this style.

The teaching style

Just as there is no such thing as a typical Australian, there is no such thing as a typical 'Carrington' teacher. But Australians do have broad characteristics that can be safely identified and so do Carrington teachers.

One of their finest qualities, arising from Mr Carrington's own personality, is the importance of making a pupil feel comfortable. The deeper meaning behind this approach is that a lesson cannot proceed when a person's fear reflexes are unduly excited. Someone who is frightened is drawn into their habitual behaviour, grasping and clinging to their familiar sense of self, and therefore finds it difficult to redirect the tension patterns that go with personality. We change best when the conditions that surround us feel supportive of taking a risk. A lesson with Walter Carrington, and many of his teachers, could be very chatty – often not related to the process of the lesson. Mr Carrington himself was a great storyteller and often span a yarn about his experiences with other pupils.

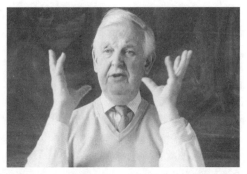

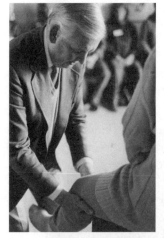

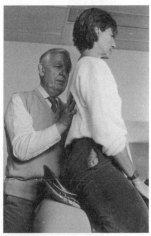

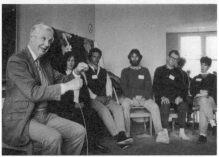

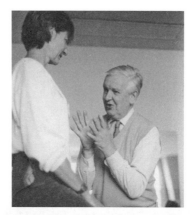

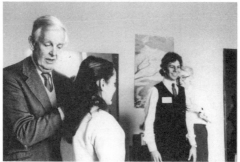

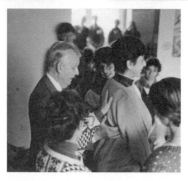

Walter Carrington: A lesson with Mr Carrington left one
with the feeling that you were very special to him. Walter
is an enthusiastic horse rider and is shown here teaching
people 'saddlework' that he personally developed for riders.

It was interesting to observe, during Mr Carrington's visit to Australia in 1989, that many of his stories seemed to be uncannily related to the background of his pupil. Was this an accident, I wondered? A musician would get a story about music, a horse rider a tale on equitation. The storytelling, I realized, became a teaching tool in itself – both giving a sense of comfort and belonging, as well as offering an embedded 'message' that acted as metaphor relating to that person's situation.

A lesson with Mr Carrington (I had many) left one with the feeling that you were special to him. It's so easy in Alexander lessons to begin feeling as if you are a mistake waiting to be fixed by the teacher. Too many teachers leave pupils with that impression of themselves. An important hallmark of the Carrington approach is to create an atmosphere of acceptance, of space and present time. As Mr Carrington explained it, it is about giving yourself time, rather than merely taking the time you need.

Critics of this style claim there is too much talk and not enough is explained – you feel wonderful at the end of a lesson, but you aren't quite sure how it was achieved or how you are supposed to regain it on your own. You begin to feel too reliant on the teacher and powerless to change by yourself. Again, be your own judge – if you feel you are learning and progressing, don't be bothered.

My understanding, as someone who has trained in this lineage (both my original teachers themselves trained with Mr Carrington), is that you are not there to have it explained! Not in so many words anyway; words of themselves are too limiting. What you are gaining is an ontological shift, a new sense of being, so how can the old you ever understand the new you? It is the nervous, dissatisfied, endlessly seeking self that wants to have it all explained, but the feeling, after a good lesson, is that all that urgency, the almost neurotic longing to be different, simply dissolves away. You become more yourself and less who you imagine yourself to be. The striving stops, the acceptance begins.

This new experience sets up a whole new way of being around others, and it is that new quality of being that the lessons are seeking to convey. You could almost say it is an ontological shift that is not related to your old way. The hungry voice that wants to ask all the questions can be just another aspect of an old way of being. How can that way of being be used to dissolve itself? You can't use your old habit to change your habit – it doesn't work that way. The critical point to seek through your lessons is self-acceptance, giving yourself space, coming into the present moment and experiencing satisfaction with yourself as you are. That is itself the point of transformation: giving up wanting to know, giving up trying, giving up being anywhere else but where you are.

The spread of teachers

Mr Carrington spent his remaining life training teachers in London after Alexander's death in 1955. So by far the greatest majority of teachers trained in this lineage live in and around London.

However, many of his teachers had, or are still running, training schools. In England there are now several training schools that follow the Carrington lineage. Also in Germany, Holland, Switzerland, Sweden, America and Australia there have been, and still are, training schools that arise from this lineage.

In Japan, where I now live, I am one of the teachers most influenced by Mr Carrington's work, as too are all the teachers I have trained. There are also a number of Japanese teachers who trained with Mr Carrington, but they have tended to remain overseas after finishing their training! Some may now be coming back – but only a few. My original training was in London in the 1970s with three teachers, Paul Collins, Elizabeth Langford and Vivien Mackie, who were all trained by Mr Carrington. When I started the school in Japan, Walter Carrington kindly wrote a personal recommendation to STAT (Society of Teachers of the Alexander Technique) in London asking them to recognize my school. This did not happen for many reasons (see 'Your teacher's qualifications' on page 106) but, until his death in 2005, Walter continued to approve of the work we are doing here and was very encouraging that we should keep it up! Vivien Mackie also visits Japan regularly at my invitation, doing many workshops for singers and musicians. Although now in her 80s, she is, like all good Alexander teachers, still enjoying remarkable health and vitality.

Patrick Macdonald (1910–1991)

A brief biography

Mr Macdonald was the son of one of Alexander's faithful supporters – Dr Peter Macdonald, a widely respected ophthalmic and aural surgeon. Dr Macdonald is famous in Alexander folklore as being one of the key movers behind a letter from 19 doctors, published in the *British Medical Journal*, calling for Alexander's discoveries to play a role in the future training of doctors. Soon after its publication in 1937, however, war broke out, quickly extinguishing this promising debate.

Like Walter Carrington, Patrick Macdonald spent his life working as an Alexander teacher, first as Alexander's first paid assistant in 1935 and then later on his own – running a training school in London and having a profound influence on the droves of Israelis who came to train with him.

He was born in York, England, in 1910 and his first contact with the work came at the age of ten, when his father – who had himself corrected a hand tremor through lessons with Alexander – decided that his son's congenital curvature of the spine needed sorting out.

The young Patrick obviously enjoyed his first lessons, as he continued them periodically until he made the fateful decision to train as a teacher of the Alexander Technique in 1932. As was the case with Mr Carrington, this was to be more to him than a simple 'profession'; it was a vocation, a passion, a lifetime's work.

While training, he is reported to have taken a leadership role in special sessions away from Alexander, where the trainees would practise hands-on and slowly develop a teaching methodology. Mr Macdonald was both an eccentric and conservative man. He prized traditional values such as discipline and responsibility while supporting many 'fringe' causes concerning environmental and conservation issues, long before they were popularized. He often left pamphlets in the waiting room for his pupils to read.

Although often criticized as a hard man, which amused him, he was capable of great acts of kindness and enjoyed a practical joke. His hardness arose out his desire for excellence: he did not suffer fools and he was his own harshest critic. When it came to his trainees, he dispensed with middle-class politeness. There was no mistaking what Mr Macdonald thought of your work.

He left London in 1937 and spent time in Birmingham, Cardiff and Brighton, building private practices and perfecting his skill. After Alexander's death in 1955, he became involved with Beaumont, Alexander's brother, and in 1957 he headed 'The Alexander Foundation' and began training teachers.

In the early 1960s, a flood of Israelis came to London and all were attracted to the no-nonsense approach and skilful teaching of Mr Macdonald. Among them were many teachers who themselves went on to found training courses in Israel, so that today the Macdonald style is almost universally adopted by teachers there.

In 1987 he fell ill – his health had been declining for several years – so he ceased directing his training school in London, which then continued on in the hands of his long-time assistant, Shoshana Kaminitz. He retired to Sussex and continued teaching until his death in 1991.

The teaching style

A lesson in the Macdonald style can be very dynamic. Mr Macdonald himself had exceptionally powerful hands and delighted in bobbing you in and out of your chair many times, often in quick succession. It was an extraordinary kind of lesson that I was lucky enough to experience from his hands in 1978. I felt myself taken to the standing position without knowing quite how he did it. Then, before I knew it, I was off down again!

'Getting yourself out of the way' or 'leaving yourself alone' is especially important. The teacher aims to guide you in a new experience and it is imperative that you 'prevent' your old habits from coming into play. It is very much an experience, in a good lesson, of the teacher doing it for you – the strong hold of their hands directing you in and out of the chair.

The lunge is also a popular procedure in lessons – one leg before the other as you then 'lunge' on to one leg, bending your knee in the process. Imagine Errol Flynn with a sword and you've got the picture. This is a cousin of 'monkey', a procedure that teachers of all lineages will at some point do with you. Monkey is the slang for Alexander's 'position of mechanical advantage' and involves bending at your hips, knees and ankles while still maintaining the full length of your back.

Perhaps the most striking feature of the Macdonald lineage is the wide practice of asking the pupil to widen their stance before getting them in and out of the chair. The feet are placed wider than the hips, very much wider in fact, so it feels more as if you are straddling the chair than sitting in it. This has proved controversial with the other teaching lineages which do not use this practice. There are photographs that show Alexander himself once worked in this way.

According to Mr Macdonald, there can be many times when this is beneficial – and certainly under his hands it worked that way – by getting a person to lengthen and widen and rise from the chair with a very different coordination from that of their habitual pattern. Critics claim it is a trick and, unless employed very skilfully, can bring about excessive strain on the legs and knees. You will have to be your own judge. Are lessons benefiting you? If they are, then don't be troubled.

Another feature – not universal, but common enough to be distinct to this lineage – is the running commentary of the teacher while they place hands on you. In this lineage there is less time for chat – your teacher will remind you of your 'Alexander directions' or 'orders' as their hands are giving you the experience of them. For example, the teacher might repeat 'Forward and up, forward and up, forward and up' almost like a mantra while their hands deliver the experience that those words imply. In that way you are trained to link the words with the experience, so that on your own the 'orders' have a stronger meaning for you and, ultimately, are more effective.

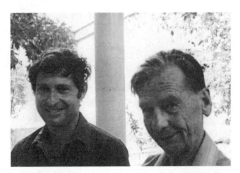

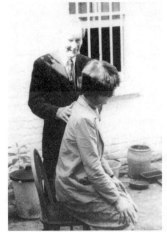

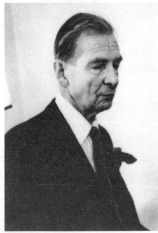

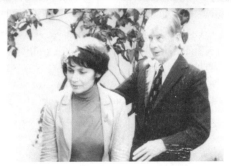

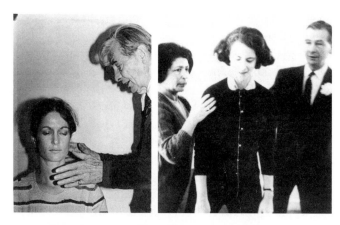

Patrick Macdonald is shown here working with
different colleagues in the later part of his life.
In Japan today there are many teachers who
can trace their lineage back to Macdonald.

The 'upthrust' is also considered of utmost importance.
'Upthrust' is the Macdonald word for lengthening but, as
the word suggests, it is considered to be a dynamic thing that
leads to movement. In this lineage, great emphasis is placed
on the 'primary control' – the head–neck relationship –
which is the source of the 'upthrust'. Another important
tenet is 'strengthening the back', which is a necessary and
natural by-product of the 'upthrust'.

Some people have likened Macdonald-type lessons to a
dance and my limited experience confirms this. It is difficult
to get bored as you are taken along for a ride by this dynamic
and active approach to Alexander's discoveries.

The spread of teachers

Most of the teachers who trained with Mr Macdonald himself
are found in London and elsewhere in England. Then, both
in England and generally the world, there is a far greater

number of second- and third-generation teachers. These are individuals trained by teachers who were themselves trained by Mr Macdonald. Being second-generation teachers, they have been more influenced by their teacher than by Mr Macdonald himself.

Looking at the rest of the world, Israel consists of almost 100 per cent Macdonald style teachers of the second-/third-generation variety. At various times there have been up to 13 training schools run by his former students in Israel. Also Switzerland, Germany and the United States have training schools arising from the Macdonald lineage. You will find teachers of this lineage in most parts of the world where Alexander teachers are to be found.

Marjorie Barstow (1899–1996)
A brief biography

Marjorie Barstow was my teacher and my friend. I was lucky enough to have retrained myself under her watchful eyes during the last ten years of her life. She was 86 when I met her and she once turned to me and declared: 'I'm so old I'm an antique!' She never took herself too seriously: 'You always move better with a smile' was her motto. Marj – as she was more affectionately known by her trainees – had the distinction of receiving the first official teacher certification ever handed out by Alexander. Of the group that commenced the training with her, she was the first to qualify; the others stayed on for another year. Not Marj. Patrick Macdonald once remarked about her: 'Oh yes. We all thought she was the best of the lot of us.'

Indeed, she went on to have one of the most influential and controversial careers of any teacher since Alexander himself.

Marjorie was born in 1899 in Ord, Nebraska, USA. Breaking with the traditional role of woman for the times

– this is middle America just after the First World War – Marj attended the University of Nebraska. She was always interested in movement, and after graduating in 1921 she began teaching ballet and ballroom dancing in a studio above her garage at home. However, soon she became dissatisfied with the progress of her students. She observed that after a certain point in their training, nothing she could teach them seemed to improve their coordination.

Here Marj picks up the story:

> 'I was in New York one summer many years ago along with my teacher studying dance. One day she came back to the apartment with an *Atlantic Monthly* in which J. Harvey Robinson had written an article called "The Philosopher's Stone." The article was about this creature, F. M. Alexander. Neither of us had heard of him, but when we finished reading the article she said, "I would like to study with that man sometime!" Well, it happened that about a year or two after that she did go to England and worked with Mr Alexander for a couple of weeks. When she came back, she brought two of his books which had been published.'

The two books were *Man's Supreme Inheritance* and *Conscious Constructive Control of the Individual.* Of these Marj declared: 'I was so fascinated with the books that I preferred to read them rather than anything else.'

In 1927, with her recently acquired movie camera underarm – Marj was always a little ahead of her time – she and her sister set forth for London. For the next six months they both had lessons every weekday – alternating between Alexander and his brother AR (Albert Reddan).

It was not long after returning from London that Marj received a letter from Alexander inviting her to return and join his first teacher training school, which she did in 1931. Three years later, in 1934, Marj returned to America.

There she spent her first six years of teaching working as AR's assistant in Boston until family circumstances necessitated Marj's return to Lincoln to take over running the family business.

The teaching style

For many years hereafter she all but disappeared from the general Alexander community in America. But Marj didn't stop working on herself. During this time she told us that she decided to 'get tough' with herself. She later often remarked that she did not really begin to understand the work until this time. It may be this period that so convinced her of the logic of applying Alexander's discoveries to all kinds of activities aside from just the applications – such as getting in and out of a chair – that Alexander had developed.

It is the widening of Alexander's original application work that is now generally recognized as one of the hallmarks of her teaching lineage. This style of application work has made itself popular with dancers, musicians and other performance-related artists who love forsaking the traditional table and chair for activities more directly related to their artistic skills.

Marj pioneered group teaching, which many teachers had considered (and still do) not a practical way to study the work effectively. Marj certainly turned that idea on its head. She began her long study of group teaching in the 1950s when the University of Nebraska invited her to teach. She continued with this work while also working in small groups with the ever-increasing flow of Alexander teachers and students making the long journey to the prairie state. Her reputation as an innovative teacher began to spread in the American Alexander community.

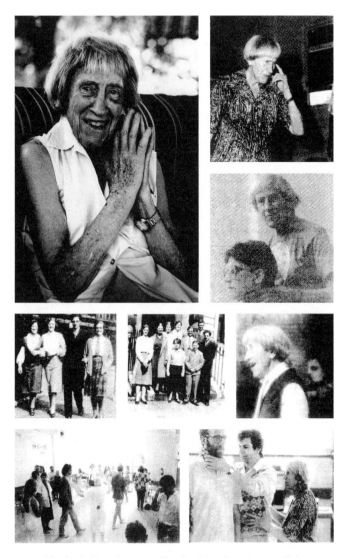

Marjorie Barstow was the first teacher to complete
Alexander's teacher training programme and taught
throughout the world until her death in 1996. The majority of
teachers in Japan today can trace their lineage back to Marj.

Her group teaching skills received a major boost in 1973 with an invitation from the Theatre Department of Southern Methodist University in Dallas, Texas, to teach Alexander's discoveries. (Marj rarely referred to the work as the Alexander Technique, preferring always to call it 'Mr Alexander's discoveries'.) The University gave little indication of what was involved and it was only upon arrival that Marj was told her class consisted of 60 people for four sessions. Rather than disappoint them, Marj proceeded to figure out a way to teach that many people at once.

Helped by her many years of experiments at the University of Nebraska, she surprised herself with the results she elicited – despite the overwhelming teacher-to-student ratio. Over the following years, as the invitations from universities, theatre centres, martial arts schools, music camps, Alexander training schools and the like flooded in, Marj began developing a methodology for group teaching that is now part of her unique teaching lineage.

A lesson with a teacher grounded in this lineage is likely to be more interactive verbally than the other lineages. It's a gross generalization which must be taken with a grain of salt, but Marj herself was always querying you in a way neither Mr Carrington or Mr Macdonald would – nor Alexander from the little I know of his teaching methods. Marj was unique in her style of teaching. Questions such as 'How does that feel?' 'What did you do just then?' 'How are you going to direct your head?' 'What do you mean by saying "floating" your head?' Some pupils loved these lessons; others felt a little confronted by them.

In the Barstow style there is also a great stock placed upon observation – both of yourself and others – which is why there is an emphasis on group teaching as opposed to the private lessons. In her later years, Marj never did table work, nor taught her trainees much about this practice, so it is less likely that you will be worked on in that way by a teacher of this lineage.

The spread of teachers

It was in Lincoln, USA, that a nucleus of serious trainees first began forming. These were people who had packed up their homes and families, left their jobs and – with no offers or guarantees of anything from Marj – moved to Lincoln to learn more from her of 'Mr Alexander's discoveries'. Only a gem of a teacher can inspire that kind of dedication: Marj had something, and those of us who were privileged enough to work with her knew it.

It was this paradoxical nature of Marj's apprenticeship-style 'not-training training' that created political tension with those in the Alexander community who had completed a formal three-year training. Marj never sought to train teachers – but neither would she deny her wisdom to the flow of hungry trainees coming to live with her in Lincoln. Flustered servants of the Alexander community began demanding of her: 'Do you train teachers?' Having never sought to do so, she authentically answered, 'No.' But then, with that cheeky glint in her eye, she would add, 'But I help people who want to be teachers.' This was a bit too Zen for the bureaucrats, and tempers and politics in the later years of her life created some lingering bad feeling in the general Alexander community about Marj's teachers.

Of course, in Japan itself I have been educating teachers since 1999. My company, BodyChance, is now the largest educator of teachers in the world. We currently have over 100 Japanese studying with us to be teachers, so Marj's work is alive and healthy in Japan!

Today, teachers of this lineage are mostly found in America, Japan, Germany and Australia, places where training programmes led by her long-time students are currently operating. In England and Europe there are almost no teachers of this lineage. Instead, you are more likely to find quite a lot of misinformation and misunderstanding. It is worth checking, if you come across any negative opinion, just how much direct experience a teacher has had. ATI, the organization mentioned previously, is where you will find the majority of teachers influenced by this Barstow lineage.

Conclusion

Of course there are many other lineages I could mention – not the least being the work of Alexander's niece, Marjory Barlow, and her husband, Dr Barlow, who together contributed enormously to the development of the work. Dr Barlow helped gain wider acceptance of the work in the performing arts and medical profession, whereas Mrs Barlow has trained many teachers. However, their trainees have not themselves started training schools – there is just one in England – so their influence and presence is not significant in relation to the three lineages I have described here.

In the end, your lesson is coming from an individual, not a lineage. Just as no one can teach as Alexander taught, also no one from any lineage will be quite the same. Individual differences can be so great as to render the 'lineage' of a teacher irrelevant. I present this information to highlight the fact that there is no such thing as the 'standard' Alexander lesson. If you are not happy at first, shop around, as there is bound to be a teacher better suited to you.

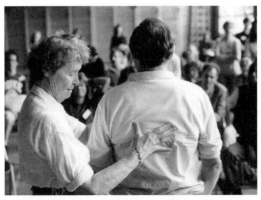

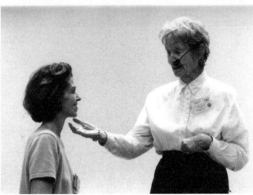

Marjory Barlow, Alexander's niece, is shown here working.
In Japan there are several third-generation teachers who
trained with teachers trained by Wilfred and Marjory Barlow.

Developments in France

In 2009 this book was translated into French and published
there. As part of that process, I collected more information
about the development of Alexander Technique in France,
and I include it here for those readers interested in the
development of Alexander's discoveries in the world.

In France, the Macdonald and Carrington lineages are most common. Most of these teachers are affiliated to the two professional organizations named previously. The number of teachers has increased with the opening of training schools in the country in the last 25 years.

One of the pioneer in France is a teacher, Marie-Françoise le Foll-Possompès. She trained in London with Patrick Macdonald in the 1970s, eventually starting the first training course in Paris in 1984. She was the Director until it ended in 1995. During that time, she invited to her school many teachers – I was one of those invited! Some of the first generation of teachers visited her school too: Dilys and Walter Carrington and Marjorie Barstow. Because of various disputes with STAT (Society of Teachers of the Alexander Technique) over the years, most of her teachers eventually became members of ATI (Alexander Technique International).

Then in 2000, at almost 80 years of age, Astrid Cox opened a training course approved by the French affiliated society, l'EFFTA (Ecole Française de Formation à la Technique Alexander). Astrid was trained in the 1970s at the same time I was at the School of Alexander Studies in Highgate, London. She comes from a Carrington lineage.

In 2005, l'EFFTA changed to L'ETAPP (Ecole de la Technique Alexander pour Professeurs à Paris), with a new director: Odyssée Gaveau. Like Marie-Françoise, Odyssée also trained in London with Macdonald a little later in the 1980s. Odyssée had been working as an assistant in several schools in England, Germany and with Marie-Françoise in Paris. She came from Sweden, where she had spent the previous ten years working privately.

6

Working with
Your Self Alone

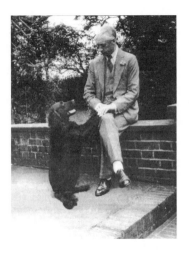

'You are not here to do exercises, or to learn to
do something right, but to get able to meet a
stimulus that always puts you wrong and to learn
to deal with it.'

F. M. Alexander

The ideas for practising on your own contained within
this chapter are procedures that I have developed for group
workshops. They are based on the ideas of the Alexander
work and aim for the same result, but they differ from
the traditional Alexander lesson. A lesson has a primary

ingredient of 'sensation' facilitated by the hands of your teacher, and this forms the basis for every other discussion, procedure and observation that goes on in a lesson. However, when working on your own, this ingredient is missing.

The question that has occupied me for most of my teaching life has been to discover how a beginner can generate an 'Alexander experience' of freedom and ease on their own, without the need of a teacher's hands. It's a radical research question because, if I successfully answered it, there'd be no need for Alexander teachers. The first two procedures that I will detail in this chapter are the processes I have developed that can, if done correctly, lead you to experience a different quality in your coordination. The third process is not my own; it is a very common procedure used by Alexander teachers, which is described in Chapter 4 under the heading 'Tablework'.

All three procedures take a different approach to the exact experimental observations in a mirror that constituted Alexander's method of observation, which is described in Chapter 7. The processes presented here are based on the model of meditation – where first you subdue your mind, then direct your thoughts along a deliberately arranged sequence of ideas. Maintaining your concentration along that sequence of thought is critical to getting positive results, so it is by no means certain that these procedures will bring any immediate benefit. Like everything worthwhile, it takes practice.

My suggestion is that you experiment with friends. It is helpful if someone can read the text while others concentrate on applying it. Alternatively, you could read the text on to an MP3 and play it back to yourself, becoming familiar with the procedure so that you can eventually dispense with it and experiment on your own.

Proprioception

Proprioception is the body's ability to sense itself. It is the key to understanding why each of these three processes works. You are learning to utilize a powerful imaging system wired into your nervous system: that of the millions of proprioceptive receptors located in every muscle, ligament and tendon of your body.

These receptors are firing off their messages continuously, but we largely suppress awareness of this input in favour of the other senses, such as seeing, hearing, smelling, tasting and touching external objects. Interestingly, all the other senses are concerned with determining our relationship with phenomena external to us. Smelling, for example, involves us actually ingesting the molecules of another substance.

Yet only one sense deals entirely with our internal universe: the proprioceptive sense. It is a miracle sense which, if accessed fully, has a wealth of previously unrealized information about ourselves. In part, the procedures I am outlining in this chapter are ways of training yourself to become sensitive to this proprioceptive sense.

The more you practise, the more natural it becomes to be mindful of your body and have an accurate awareness of your coordination. This benefit will eventually extend to activities such as walking, bending and all the other things you do in a day. So, now you are sitting quietly, you are ready to begin using this proprioceptive sense to map your primary holding pattern.

Remaining still

All three of these processes require that you remain still for a period of time, just as you would do if you were meditating. You decide how long, but ten minutes is sufficient to start.

Why is that so many people dread the idea of staying still? Alternatively, you could ask: why is it we fidget and move around all the time? Watch yourself right now. Are you remaining quietly still as you read or are you shaking your foot, fiddling with your hair, chewing gum, biting your lip, holding your legs unnecessarily tight or grabbing on with something else? If you observe yourself carefully, you will find that you are doing something which, upon honest analysis, isn't really necessary. Why is that?

Sometimes I play a little game with myself. In a cafe I pick someone and watch this constant movement, observing how it transforms itself into different actions from one moment to the next: first my subject is tapping his fingers; then he stops that and crosses his legs and, for a second, does nothing; then he starts fiddling with the salt on the table until he lights up a cigarette and puffs away on that. Then he...

This activity never stops – always, always, always there is some sort of fidgeting going on. Human 'beings' is the wrong name for us; we should call ourselves human 'doings'. We so often experience this underlying restlessness which manifests itself into small, seemingly insignificant, but nevertheless unrelenting activities.

Stop these activities. Just remain still and quietly watch yourself. Try it now as you read. Can you do it? There is a primary motivation for all this fidgeting: it is an attempt to 'get away' from yourself, from some feeling of discomfort or agitation. Analyze a few of the fidgeting actions. Why do you do them? What is the impulse, the need that the movement answers within you? Is it a seeking, a wanting-of-something, directing each movement?

Making these actions all the time serves to distract you from experiencing your underlying condition. When you do stop and experience that condition, it can be quite overwhelming within a minute. Dizziness, nausea, fear and nervousness are not uncommon initial experiences. I've had pupils declare that they couldn't do it – they just couldn't stay still, not even for a minute – and get angry at the idea that I am asking them to. Also, for a few people, it feels blissful, a relief to stop in this way. Your experience will probably fall somewhere between these two extremes.

Primary holding pattern

Step 1: Self-acceptance

There is a deeper meaning to this first step of becoming still and that is to accept yourself. Be comfortable with being uncomfortable. Give up trying to make things 'better'. Embrace yourself with all your 'imperfections'. It isn't possible to make changes against a background of denial.

Denial, in this case, means trying not to be who you are being. Most of your postural adjustments are made against a background of wanting to get rid of some discomfort. It is as though you are using the discomfort to push yourself somewhere else – and there's the irony. In order to push, you need something to push on, so no matter how hard you try to get away from your discomfort, you always need it to do the getting away. Alexander said:

'Trying is only emphasizing the thing we already know.'

It's a Catch-22 situation: you want to get away from your discomfort but you have to use it to get away, so it always goes with you. This is simple to understand: if you weren't slumping, why would you need to sit up? What happens after you have sat up for a while? Figure 6.1 shows how this progresses – eventually, you slump down worse than ever.

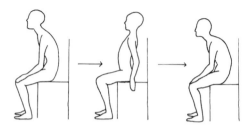

Figure 6.1 When we find ourselves slumping, first we make
a tremendous effort to hold ourselves up, but after a while
we tire of that and then slump down worse than ever.

Self-acceptance is paradoxically a way of escaping from
this never-ending cycle. You learn to stop seeing yourself
as a mistake waiting to be fixed and move deeper into your
feelings of discomfort. Instead of fighting yourself, you start
to tolerate yourself, even feel love and compassion towards
yourself.

During the first minutes of remaining quiet, the urges to
move don't stop. Observe them with indifference, each time
freshly making a decision: 'No, I won't make that movement;
I will continue to remain quiet and still within my body and
accept these conditions as they are.' If you keep working on
this premise of accepting yourself, a strange thing can start
to happen: it becomes easier, almost pleasurable, to remain
this way. When your mind has quietened to the point where
you no longer feel urges to keep adjusting some part of your
body, then you are ready to move on to the next step of each
procedure.

In the beginning you may never get beyond this first
step. That's fine: it is better to take the time to calm your
mind than proceed in an agitated state.

Step 2: Mapping your primary holding pattern

This second step involves sensing the primary holding pattern of your musculature. You are going to be mapping the activity of the 'being' muscles associated with your motor hold system. See the headings 'Motor hold and motor move' and 'Being and doing muscles' in Chapter 3 to review this point. Motor hold is the pattern formed by the deep, intrinsic 'being' musculature that maintains your integrity during movement. It is your personality's signature and a reservoir of unexpressed emotion. Expect to occasionally experience strong emotions as you continue practising this procedure.

You don't begin with emotions, however; you begin practically by slowing mapping out the relative spatial relationships between different parts of your body. To do this procedure, pick a common, everyday posture. I suggest you use sitting in a chair as that is something we all do. Take a position that you consider comfortable rather than trying to sit correctly. Read the section under the heading 'The preliminary stance' in Chapter 7 for a fuller explanation of this. When you have achieved a degree of quiet as outlined in Step 1 above, move to the body mapping described below. This procedure can be done in any position; however, I will write with the assumption that you are sitting back in a chair.

Your left and right shoulder-arms

Arms don't end at the shoulder: your shoulder is just part of your arm. If you were a bird, the 'arm' part has all the feathers on it, whereas the 'shoulder' part is where all the muscle power and movement of the arm is anchored. To get around this crazy division that language makes, I will call it the shoulder-arm.

Compare your two shoulder-arms. Which is tighter? If you are not sure, just leave your attention on them both and wait. A stronger impression of your shoulder-arms will emerge. The 'waiting' gives you time to discern the subtle proprioceptive feedback that is coming from these two shoulder-arms. Part of this practice is learning to become more sensitive to proprioceptive feedback – the 'lost sixth sense', according to Dr Garlick at the University of New South Wales. Eyesight and hearing overwhelm proprioception, so we have little experience of being able to discriminate all the subtleties that are available to us within this proprioceptive sense.

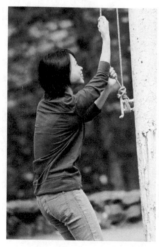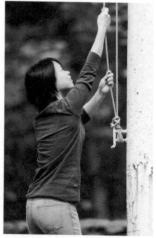

These two images demonstrate the dramatic difference the use of your shoulder-arm will have on the coordination of your whole movement. Photos by Akihiro Tada.

Ask yourself: do my shoulders feel exactly the same? This is next to impossible. Then ask: how are they different? Keep creatively sensing them both – the top, the bottom, the inside and the outside of everything you consider to be a 'shoulder'.

Now begin orientating their position in space relative to each other. Which is higher? Which is further forward? Again, wait until a definite impression emerges. Often it won't become immediately apparent but, after time, you will gain a clearer impression. You may have felt that you started in a straight position, but as you go in you might find you are more like the person in Figure 6.2. Once you have a clear impression, move on.

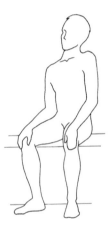

Figure 6.2 This shows an exaggerated version of the slight twists that we hold our body in most of the time – the head cocks to one side, one of the shoulders is held back and down, or the torso is twisted around and one of our legs turns out more than the other. Check yourself right now.

Your head and neck

Just where does your shoulder-arm end and your neck begin? Of course, this is an impossible question because there is no exact place. So – widen the sense of your shoulder-arm to include the two sides of your neck. It is important in this process of mapping your holding pattern that you build upon the previous mapping you have done. In this case, retain the impression of your shoulder-arms as you begin mapping the head and neck.

Which side of your neck feels tighter? Does this relate to the shoulder-arm that is tighter? Can you feel how it is continuous, all the same tension? As with the shoulder-arm, transform this feeling of tension into a spatial orientation: which side of the neck feels shorter? Are you leaning your head more to one side? How does this fit in with what you are experiencing with your shoulder-arms? Again, take time until a clear impression of your shoulder-arms and head leaning emerges.

Your rib cage and pelvis

Now sense the contact of your back against the chair. While still maintaining an awareness of your shoulder-arms, neck and head, check which side of your back has more contact or pressure against the back of the chair? Are you making contact with the back of the chair with the same or different areas of your back? Can you relate that to your shoulders and head and neck and make sense of it as part of a whole pattern of holding?

Check the two sides of your rib cage – between the bottom ribs and the top of the pelvis bone on the two sides of your body. Do these two sides feel as long as each other or does it feel as if one side is shorter because your rib cage is compressed down more on one side? Again, relate this to everything you are sensing with the head, neck, shoulder-arms and back and see if it all fits together into a pattern of holding.

Now sense the contact your sitting bones have with the chair. Are you right on them or sitting on the back part of your bottom? Is the pressure equal on both sides or can you feel more on one side than the other? Does this follow from what is happening to the rest of your body? Is it fitting into an overall pattern?

Your legs, knees and feet

While still retaining the overall impression of your body built up to now, join to it the awareness of your two legs. Particularly sense the position of your knees relative to each other: is one pulled in more than the other? Alternatively, does one knee feel more opened out than the other? Can you feel how this is a result of the whole primary holding pattern through your body; that the position of your head, shoulders, rib cage and pelvis all combine to cause your two legs to be in the position they are in?

Finally, with this overall awareness, check out your feet and how they are placed on the floor – if indeed they are both on the floor. Which part of your foot has more pressure on it? Are you collapsing the foot inwards into the arch or turning it outwards and lifting the arch of the foot? Can you understand this movement relative to the position of your knees and the body above it? Again, figure out how it fits in with the whole pattern from head down. With practice, this whole stage can be done in as little as a few seconds. Even less. Remember, the information is always there; learning to listen and interpret it is all you're practising to do.

Step 3: Making the parts whole

By now it will become clearer that you are twisting your body a little to the left or the right – this is almost universally true. Keep up the questions, being creative and thinking of your own, until a clear impression of a whole body twist begins to emerge. If initially you can't discern a twist, keep up the questions and your patience until an impression finally emerges.

Often this impression arrives in a sudden flash. I have often seen the look of surprise on a student's face as all the disparate aches and pains in different areas of their body suddenly make sense to them – an outcome of one holistic twist through the body. This Step 3 is the point you were working towards in Step 2, to 'realize' that you are holding yourself in an overall twist from the top of your head to the tip of your feet.

I cannot go into the hundreds of different ways you can go about mapping this pattern; it is for you to take this blueprint and start to work creatively on your own. The astute reader will realize that in the foregoing I have only guided you through mapping an overall rotational twist. I did this in part because rotation can include within it all other movements of the body (flexion, extension, abduction, adduction, lateral flexion and extension and other, more specialized movement patterns).

However, it is also possible to analyze each movement category separately. For example, you may decide to examine at first only whole-body flexion (bending your body forward in a slump-like fashion) and extension (arching your body back). This can be quite useful to understanding how the action of the head and neck is integral to causing downward pressure through your whole body.

Beginner's mind

It is important that your impression of this overall holding pattern arises by itself, that it isn't an intellectual imposition on your body arising from abstract notions you may currently entertain or according to what some expert told you. Even if they are right, you still have to experience it within your body. Truly understanding is feeling, not just a dry, intellectual knowing. If done correctly, this procedure definitely gives you the feeling of discovering something that was there all the time but hidden from your awareness. It is important not to think you know already what you are doing before you start, even if you have practised this process a hundred times. A story of my teacher Marj illustrates this point.

Once Marj and I were on a walk around the coastline of Sydney harbour. She was tired, so she sat herself on a bench looking out to sea while I was exploring a mysterious set of steps leading down to the shore. When I returned and sat down beside her, she looked at me and remarked, 'Do you know what I was doing while you were down there?'

'No, Marj,' I said, 'I do not.'

'Well,' she answered, 'I was just trying to figure out what "forward and up" was.'

As the reader will know by now, 'forward and up' is the fundamental Alexander direction, the first thing you learn in a lesson. So here was Marj, now a teacher of over 50 years, still trying to figure it out! Of course, Marj's lesson for me – she was a crafty old fox who understood exactly how I tended to distract my observations with theories all the time – was to remind me never to assume anything, not to entertain the arrogant notion that I already know. Shunryu Suzuki, a Zen master from Japan, wrote: 'In the beginner's mind there are many possibilities, but in the expert's mind there are few.'

Every time you experiment with this procedure, approach it with a beginner's mind.

Step 4: Going in further

Now you have gained this holistic awareness of your primary holding pattern, it is time to play with it a little, to develop your relationship to this pattern. There are several alternative strategies to take in exploring further this primary holding pattern. You can try them out one after the other, or each one alone during any one session.

First, remain sensing the holding pattern in a non-linear way. Let me explain. Previously, you have built up an impression step by step, moving through your body from the top down. Your attention has been deliberately directed along certain lines. Now, let your attention be free to roam where it wants to. This still means focusing on the body, not drifting off into unrelated daydreaming, but there is no order to it, no logic in it. Your attention 'does itself', so to speak. This can deepen your perception of your whole holding pattern, revealing previously unrecognized aspects of it. Be intuitive: go with what suggests itself.

Second, it is useful to accentuate the holding pattern. Twist more in the direction you feel you are already going in. Do this very delicately, with great awareness of the whole pattern throughout the process of exaggerating it. Determine where you make the effort. Which muscle groups seem to be engaged to exaggerate your holding? Does the exaggerated movement increase the strain you feel at different places in your body? Where? Can you feel if it starts in a particular place or does it happen as a whole? Is more work done in one place compared to another?

Third, experience the emotional charge of your holding pattern. Feel it as an attitude – a way you have of relating to the world, a communication you are making to others about yourself. Are you accepting, fighting or withdrawing from the world? Or are you pulling away with one part, pushing against with another? Do you feel weak or strong? Is there a sadness set within you, or frustration and irritation, even anger?

Simply let these impressions emerge of their own accord. The act of focusing attention is enough. If nothing emerges, don't force it. Revisit this again another time.

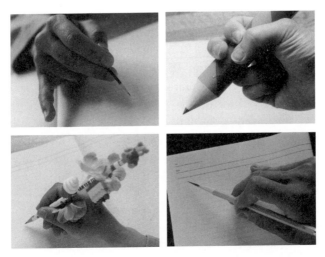

Everyone can hold a pencil, but no two pencils are the same. How we use ourselves is like that – something is similar, but something is very different too. Photos by Akihiro Tada.

Step 5: Personalized directions

As I have explained previously, our usual attempts to 'correct' a feeling of tension and discomfort normally involves us going 'against' the tension spot, as in making an effort to 'sit up' against the tendency to slump. The difference in this approach is that we are going into our tension, embracing it, coming to know it intimately and, through that process, letting the holding pattern simple dissolve away. Marj used to teach us: 'All you'll get is the absence of what you had.'

If you have followed the previous steps carefully, this step needs no explanation. Once you fully realize the extent of your holding pattern, 'releasing' does itself. It's as though you wake up to all the holding you are doing and, because you sense it so clearly, there is nothing to figure out any more – releasing it is obvious. If you can't release easily, it is axiomatic that you haven't seen your pattern clearly and you need to repeat Steps 1 to 4 more thoroughly. However, there are some pointers worth bearing in mind during this next step.

First, the key to any undoing of tension is to reverse the direction of the contraction by allowing your body to unravel in exactly the opposite direction. Notice the words 'allowing' and 'unravel'. The point is to release by lengthening the muscles that are shortening and pulling you down, rather than engage other muscles to pull you up. Remember, lengthening a muscle means releasing it. All a muscle can do is contract.

Second, most techniques of relaxation miss this point. It is not enough to tell a muscle to 'relax'; they don't respond too well to that, do they? What you must know is *the direction to think it in* to release it. If you are pulling to the left, then the only way to 'relax' those muscles is to release them towards the right. Dropping more to the left will only increase the stress you have.

Third, these become your new personalized Alexander directions. You can begin to think of them at other times of the day, always relating them back to the holding pattern they release. These directions are not along the lines of 'head forward and up, back lengthen and widen, knees forward and away' that I describe later, in Chapter 7. Instead, they are directions unique to you, based on a clear perception of how you are holding yourself. If you keep up this practice, they will keep changing every time. What works for a few days won't work for ever. Keep them fresh by returning to this process of delicate, patient observation and rediscovering again and again the coordinated pattern of holding you have.

Fourth, as you 'unravel' your holding pattern, using your personalized directions, expect it to feel strange, even wrong. Also expect to suddenly release the aches and tension you feel. If you don't experience that, you are being too forceful.

This is the key moment: if you have done well, and move delicately, now's the time you get results. Your experience can parallel the effect of a teacher's hands-on work with you. It is a sweet moment and worth all the effort, because this experience can stay with you for days. You have engineered your personal Alexander directions.

Step 6: Exploring the critical moment

Up until now you have only investigated the intrinsic, muscular holding pattern. Although it is vital, it isn't the whole story. Layered over this holding pattern, and interacting and affecting it, are the larger, grosser, extrinsic muscle groups that are responsible for the bigger movements of walking, bending, using the arms and legs and so on. (Review the section under the heading 'Motor hold and motor move' in Chapter 3 for expansion on this point.) How do these bigger movements affect your primary holding pattern? Alternatively, how does your primary holding pattern affect these bigger movements?

A simple movement to pick for answering these questions is that of moving forward in the chair. Start back in the chair and go through all the previous steps, up to and including the release of your primary holding pattern. At this time consider the idea of moving forward in the chair. Immediately you think that thought, observe the result in your body. Research has shown that merely the thought of a movement causes activity in the musculature that will eventually perform that movement. Your aim is to reach a degree of sensitivity so that you can detect these subtle changes before you actually move. At the very moment you detect yourself tensing, release out of the decision to move and go back to just sitting again.

Spend a lot of time dancing between beginning to move forward in the chair and then releasing by deciding against this action. Both times – the decision to move and the decision to stop – have to be genuine. The intention has to be honest and not a ruse for observation. As you observe this dance around the critical moment of action/non-action, you can analyze all the preparatory movements you make to move forward from the chair.

How do these preparatory movements compare to your habitual primary holding pattern? Do you feel yourself going back into the pulls and tightening that you just spent ten minutes thinking yourself out of? This step is another useful way of giving you an impression of your primary holding pattern. Using this step and the previous ones, you can explore it thoroughly – first in stillness, then in activity.

Now comes the interesting part. Can you move forward in the chair without going back into your habitual holding pattern? It should feel very strange to even attempt to do this. Your feelings, being unfamiliar with this kind of coordination, will baulk at any attempt to move this way. There will be an overwhelming feeling that you have to pull down in the way you are accustomed to in order to move forward in the chair.

Decide anyway that you won't move forward. Instead, give your personalized directions and, while continuing to project those to your body, move forward in the chair. How did you go? Check it out. Have you pulled back into your habitual holding pattern at all? Did the moving forward from the chair feel easier than usual or did it feel stiff?

You have to be very honest with yourself at this point. We all love to succeed, but the truth is you are most likely to have failed. The failure, in fact, is the basis of success, of learning. Expect it, embrace it and reconsider what you have done and experiment again. The most common fault for a beginner at this time is to brace and stiffen yourself by trying to hold yourself in a new position while you move forward from the chair. If that happens, you will feel robotic. However, don't be discouraged – this happens to pupils in lessons all the time. Be patient and kind with yourself. Keep experimenting along the lines I have suggested. This is a long-term process, not a quick fix.

Sensing sub-occipital muscles

The sub-occipitals are a group of muscles that are vitally important and, through experiments with myself and my pupils, I have discovered that they have an uncanny and disproportionate influence on our entire coordination. There is no substantial scientific evidence that I can find to support this idea, other than the remarkable and unique physiological profile of these muscles. However, if you follow this mediation faithfully, you will be rewarded with experiential, empirical evidence of the efficacy of this idea. Science might take another century – don't wait.

Profile of the sub-occipital muscles

The most finely controlled muscles in the human body are those that manipulate our eyes. The second most finely controlled muscles are those that move our tongue. Both of these are to be expected – no surprise. But the third group in this category? The sub-occipital muscle group – have you even heard of them? Could you account for why they have been endowed with such remarkable powers of control? Just who are these sub-occipital muscles and why are they there?

See Figure 6.3 for locating the sub-occipital and other related muscles. The 'sub' is for below, like subway train; the 'occipital' is the name of the bone they attach to, which forms the base of the skull. Anatomically, not all the muscles shown in Figure 6.3 are included in the sub-occipital group,

but it is easier from now on to refer to all of them by
that name.

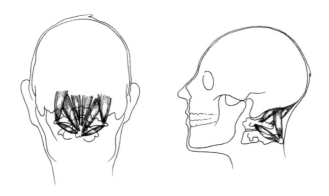

Figure 6.3 The location of the sub-
occipital and other related muscles.

If you look at the two diagrams in Figure 6.3, what should
be obvious is that these muscles don't have the strength or
leverage to move the head around. Our head is too heavy
for these muscles to take its weight; other larger, stronger
muscles take the weight of the head and make its movements.
So, strictly speaking, the sub-occipitals can't even perform as
muscles!

Step 1: Primary control

Alexander's 'primary control' concept will be covered
in greater detail in Chapter 7. As you will discover in
that chapter, the sub-occipital muscles sound remarkably
synchronous with this function dreamed up by Alexander.
To be fair to Alexander, he never thought of the 'primary
control' as a sensory 'thing', in the way that an ear or an
eye is a sensory thing. He stated that it only exists in the

'sphere of relativity', by which he means it arises out of a relationship between various 'things'.

This makes sense in relation to the sub-occipital muscles. The one thing they can do, and do very well, is act as detectors of the subtle movements of the head as it balances on top of the spine. They are both the position detectors and movers of the head's relation to the spine. I think of them as being like the power-steering device of a car – they effortlessly control the powerful muscles underneath them to correct and align our little dance of coordination.

Step 2: Sub-occipital muscle activity

First, make this observation. Watch the head of several friends as they are standing or sitting still. At first glance it will appear that their head is still. But, similar to letting your eyes adjust to the dark, let your eyes adjust to seeing tiny movements and then it will become apparent that, actually, the head never stops moving. Ask your friend to stop moving their head and they will ask you what are you talking about – to them their head is still. They can't feel these tiny movements, yet you can clearly see them happening.

The first aim of this process is for you to gain such a level of sensitivity that you can feel this constant wobbling about of your head. Before you start, study Figure 6.3 and practise visualizing the actual location in your body of these different muscles. Work towards developing a clear and accurate imagery of them.

Reread the section titled 'Remaining still' at the start of this chapter. Having prepared yourself in this way, begin by resting your attention on the area of the sub-occipital muscles. Actually, that's all you ever have to do, but it will become unbearable for some. One of several things will happen first.

First, you could feel nothing – find it almost impossible to let your attention dwell at that area because it feels numb or non-existent to you. It might feel as though I am asking you to be aware of a door knob in the room – it seems meaningless and impossible to achieve. If that's the first result you get, then you need to be doing this process! It is a sign that you are way out of touch with this important muscle group.

Second (or this could be your first experience), you feel this area as tight, extremely tense – almost unbearably so. You could feel that you want to move your head or do something. This is a good sign. By resting your attention, you are not so much making more tension as you are waking up to the tension you already have. My own experience with these muscles is that they are normally in a chronic state of perpetual contraction and, until you can directly perceive this condition consciously, it isn't possible to bring about any release. At this stage, this area feels like a big, thick, unmoving block of hard, aching tension.

Third (again this could be your first experience), you feel the activity of this muscle group. This is an advanced state of awareness that you are aiming for: now you are actually sensing all the little movements of the head that you have observed others doing. It is only when you reach this stage that you can start the important process of talking to these muscles, quietening them down, bringing your head to an increasingly still but poised condition. However, before you start with that, just spend time becoming familiar with that constant activity. Listen to it, feel how your head is moving, visualize the activity in each of the muscles. The activity of the sub-occipital muscles can feel like an uncontrollable twitch – you observe something happening without the feeling that you are making it happen.

Step 3: Discerning differences

Start to discern differences between the different directions of movement – that is, forward and backward, side to side and twists to the left or right. Continuous observation will reveal that one side is busier than the other – that your head leans to a favoured side. Keep on sensing until you can make this discernment. Actually, there is no end to increasing your sensitivity to these muscles. There is always more movement to sense, and the seeing of it makes the food that the observation feeds upon.

If you like, you can move straight on to Step 4 below, or you can experiment further. Revisit the activities laid out in 'Step 5: Personalized directions' in the 'Primary holding pattern' process described previously. This can form the basis of further experiments.

Step 4: Moving around

The oddest part of this process is that you often won't experience the full benefits of this process until you start to move around again. Start by turning your head gently from side to side. How does it feel? If you've followed the instructions carefully, you will be rewarded with an easier, freer-feeling movement. Now get up and walk around a little. How does walking feel? Are you noticing any difference?

My experience is that it will never feel the same twice. Also, the longer you can tolerate just sitting there, letting your attention abide at the location of the sub-occipitals, the more you become able to generate quite powerful experiences of release in unexpected parts of your body. It is by no means restricted to the area of your head and neck.

Semi-supine procedure

Most Alexander lessons will at some point involve you lying flat on your back, with books under your head and your knees pointing up. It is called the semi-supine position as shown in Figure 6.4. Why do this?

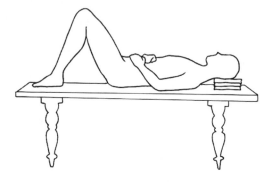

Figure 6.4 The semi-supine position for constructive rest.

First, semi-supine is a position that engineers your spine to be at maximum rest, allowing its curves to lengthen and assisting a releasing of the intrinsic, being muscles of your spine. These being muscles are mostly in an unnecessarily tight and contracted state. See 'Being and doing muscles' in Chapter 3.

Second, the intervertebral discs of your spine, which are under considerable pressure while you are upright, have a chance to rejuvenate themselves. In simplistic terms, discs sit in between each vertebrae to act as shock absorbers for your spine. In the normal course of the day, these discs are slowly compressed by the pressure of weight-bearing – you literally shrink a little every day. At night you grow again: these vertebrae expand by absorbing the fluids that surround them rather like a sponge, ready for the next day. However, 16 hours is a long wait and it enhances the health of your discs if you give them a chance to 'sponge up' once or twice during the day by lying in semi-supine.

Third, semi-supine offers an opportunity to organize your musculature by thinking through your Alexander directions while in a passive and undemanding position of coordination. It beats slumping in a chair when you get home. Alexander teachers call it constructive rest.

Getting into semi-supine

It is worthwhile getting down into semi-supine thoughtfully. Taking time to arrive in the position with a little length is vastly superior to getting down hurriedly and ending up contracted, twisted and generally shortened through your body. Look at Figure 6.5, which shows a beneficial method of getting down on to to the floor in semi-supine.

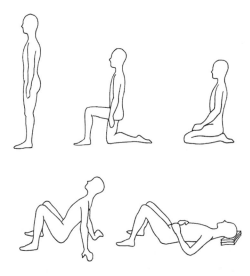

Figure 6.5 Stand at the correct distance from the books and follow this procedure to get down on to the floor. Taking time with this step makes the whole process more beneficial.

Once there, take a note of these points.

First, place some books under your head. There are different schools of thought in the Alexander world as to how many books it is best to place under your head. As a rough guide, stand yourself against a wall so that just your shoulder blades and buttocks are lightly touching it. Stand looking ahead and ask someone to measure the distance between the back of your head and the wall. This is a crude measure, so use it as a starting point only. Experiment with different heights till you find one that feels neither too high (tucking your chin in too close to your neck) nor too low (feeling that your head is falling back) but seems comfortable for you.

The aim is to bring your head to a height that leaves it in as neutral a relation to the rest of the spine as it would be when standing and looking straight ahead. Use books, not a cushion, because they give your head a firm contact, stopping it from sinking backwards as it would if you used a cushion. If your head presses too hard and feels uncomfortable, use a towel to soften the contact, but still make sure it is a firm surface. Your neck should be free of any contact with the books.

Second, the reason your knees are bent up is to take pressure off your lower back. If you find it difficult to keep your legs up – some people find they keep falling outwards – you could place some large cushions under each knee and rest your legs on them. Some people place a chair underneath the lower half of their legs, but that will only work if the chair is roughly equal to the height of your knees.

Check your lower back: is it in contact with the floor or is there still an arch? Of course, you could lift your pelvis and tuck in your bottom to flatten out your lower back against the floor, but this goes against the Alexander principle of 'non-doing' explained in Chapter 3. Don't do that.

Instead, get down again, this time watching to see that you don't arch your back in as you unroll your torso down on to the floor. If there's still an arch, leave it. With time and practice, this arch will level to make contact with the floor. And maybe it never will because your back is built that way. It's hard to give directions that apply to everyone.

Third, your arms are best placed on your torso where they feel easy and comfortable. For some people, this may mean on your hips; for others, on your tummy. Experiment a little to find out what seems natural. However, don't hold your hands together – it is better that they don't touch. This assists you in becoming aware of each separately and avoids creating unnecessary tension from holding your hands together.

Some teachers like their pupils to place their hands beside their body rather than on it, with the palms faced down to the floor roughly at the level of your lower back. Try it if you like – maybe you prefer that.

So, now you're there, what do you do next?

How not to think

Listen, sense and observe your body before projecting any messages to release it. Too many techniques are having us immediately 'doing' things – either literally by exercise, however subtle or gentle that might be, or figuratively, by imagining waterfalls or blue light or just telling muscles to relax, be heavy and the like. Please, don't start that way.

Instead, take the time to get to know your tension well. Become its friend and then you'll be able to understand it. While you are always pushing it away, trying to get rid of it, what hope have you of really understanding what you do to make this tension?

Start by simply 'being' with yourself. Just being – not trying to fix, make better, correct or adjust anything. Instead, just listen, sense, observe. Open the space of your body by giving time for your thoughts. Quit the feeling of being in a hurry. Instead, give yourself time, lots and lots of time, and let the process unfold at its own pace without you trying to force things along.

How to think

Ponder this fact: right now, as you lie in semi-supine, there are millions upon millions of messages being created by the countless sensory nerve endings in your body. This staggering body of information is continually arriving to be processed by your brain, but this normally happens below the level of conscious awareness. So open yourself to becoming aware of all these subtle vibrations and movements that are happening continuously. Just being with the sensations of your body as they arise is enough; this by itself leads you to understand what will be useful to 'direct' into your body when it comes time to do that.

As an example, I will go through how to think about your head and neck area. Use this same method to explore the different areas of your body. Generally, it is good to begin with your head and neck, then progress down your torso (ribs and pelvis) and arms (shoulders, elbows and hands) and finally to the legs (hips, knees and feet).

Muscles are organized around joints, so, as a general guide, it is useful to centre your awareness around joints. Buy yourself a simple anatomy book and check where they are located. Many muscles will have one joint as their focal point. By sensing the activity around that joint, you can sense the pulls and contractions of a large number of muscles.

By example: head and neck area

Start by becoming aware of your head and neck. Locate the joints where sub-occipital muscles operate at base of your skull. These are explored in depth in the 'Sub-occipital muscles' process. Just letting your awareness dwell in this area will slowly allow sensations to emerge; you become aware of activity, even stiffness. At that point, you can project messages to ease and calm the activities you sense happening.

Another useful way of becoming aware of an area is to sense the points of contact that, in this case, your head and shoulders make with the floor. Simply feel the weight bearing down at these points. Take in the fact that your neck is suspended between these points of contact. How does it feel to you?

Notice if your awareness is superficial or deep. Do you just think of the skin area? Practise sensing in volumes – length, breadth and height. Specifically, which areas feel tight or stiff? Where is your awareness dim? Is there a particular spot that is tense or stiff? If so, explore it further. Where does the 'stiffness' end? How superficial or deep is the feeling? Follow the sensation of 'stiffness' until you begin to appreciate that the 'stiffness' is actually part of a whole holding pattern of your neck and not only a specific pain in one small location. Again, with this awareness it becomes easier to give 'directions' to the area for it to lengthen and release.

Thinking in activity revisited

When lying in semi-supine, it is important that you apply Alexander's principle of 'thinking in activity'. See the same heading in Chapter 2. In practice, this means that as you explore sensations in your body, you expand your attention to become more inclusive. For example, as you bring an awareness to your torso, continue with the awareness of your head and neck. Practise understanding the links, the continuity between the two areas. How does one connect into the next?

While it can be useful now and again to experiment with laser-like attention – focusing on one especially tight area to the exclusion of all else – it is generally going to be more effective if you work to explore the connections that surround that area. This is partly what is meant by thinking in activity. A really sore lower back, for instance, tends to draw your attention to it, yet the real culprit could be the way your legs are pulling on your lower back, or the way your chest is puffing up in the air.

By thinking in activity and collecting together the awareness of several areas all together, one after the other, there is a greater chance that you will magically hit upon a pattern of holding that you had previously been unaware of. By understanding the holistic operation of your coordination, you have a better chance of unmasking the patterns that create unnecessary tension.

Creative thinking

On a base of self-awareness, it is fun to be creative with abstract images – I am not against that. My point is that you must include an awareness of simply being. Start with a mind that is listening/sensing/observing before you plunge into wildly creative imagery. With awareness, creative thinking can be fantastic for opening up your body and mind, but, without awareness, it easily becomes delusional and distorts our perception.

An example of this positive creativity would be to feel that the weight of your body is supported, not just by the floor or the building you are in, but the whole of Mother Earth. You have an entire planet supporting your body;

there's no need to hold on any more. Visualize the planet you are on, then give over your weight to her, fall into the arms of Mother Earth.

It is also true that above, beyond the ceiling, is space, infinite space, stretching beyond anything we can understand. Mystery surrounds us every second of our lives, but our minds are mostly contracted and closed off from this wondrous infinity that exists around our bodies every second we breathe. Take it in. Imagine that your mind has no boundaries and can fill this space. If you can imagine yourself in a faraway place, why not imagine your mind expanding to fill the entire universe?

7

The Anatomy
of Moving

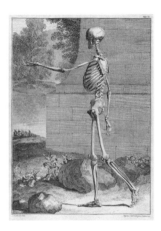

'When anything is pointed out, our only idea is
to go from wrong to right in spite of the fact
that it has taken years to get wrong: we try to get
right in a moment.'

F. M. Alexander

I have left this chapter until last as, unlike the rest of the
book, it is not really a chapter to read – it is a workbook.
If you are interested in working on your own, I've written
this chapter for you. Practise the process described in the
'Primary holding pattern' section in Chapter 6 before
embarking on all these experiments. It is vital that you train

yourself in the use of your proprioceptive (internal imaging) sense before embarking on these experiments, which favour eyesight.

These experiments are along the lines that Alexander himself followed. Most of the quotes come from the chapter 'Evolution of a Technique' in Alexander's *The Use of the Self*. I recommend you read his book if you like to be thorough.

Some Alexander teachers won't like that I am presenting this information at all, mainly because they feel concerned that you will confuse or even harm yourself – and they have a point. I can't guarantee that you won't, but I also know there are many people who can't get to a teacher and feel frustrated that most Alexander books never give precise instructions about how to experiment with this work. After all, as Alexander himself was quoted as saying:

> 'Anyone can do what I do if they will do what I did. But none of you want the discipline.'

These experiments require discipline and a lot of patience. They require time and a willingness to experience confusion, frustration and failure. After all, Thomas Edison failed thousands of times before he succeeded in inventing the light bulb. The nature of experimentation is to fail; once you succeed, what is there to experiment about? But if you persevere, the light will come on.

The Alexander directions

There are four Alexander 'directions'.

At least, that's the Alexander jargon name for what you'll learn when you take lessons to retrain your coordination. In this chapter I will explore the first two of them.

There are two aspects to 'giving directions'. The first, and most important, is the *quality of the thinking*: are you being delicate or pushy? This has been discussed at length in Chapter 3. The second aspect of this thinking is *what you actually think*: in what direction do you think of your body parts going? That is what this chapter is about. I am going to help you discover the thinking required for the first two directions. That is ambitious. Not many readers will follow through even that far. After all, it took Alexander many years while working on his own, so I doubt you can do it any quicker.

For that reason, let me issue a *caveat emptor* about these experiments.

First, the assumption underlying all these experiments is that I already know how you are misusing yourself, and, really, how can I know that? Maybe you don't pull your head back and down – I've met maybe three people who didn't. What I have done is draw upon my many years of teaching experience to illustrate what one teacher calls the 'classic downward pull' that most of us make. Notice the word 'most'. It doesn't mean 'all'. Maybe you're the exception. Then, a lot of what I have written here will be meaningless to you. So, if that's the case, sorry. It's a risk I take and a limitation of the written word.

Second, if you experiment on your own with the information in this chapter, while disregarding the necessity to monitor the delicacy of your thinking and movements, then you will do yourself harm. No question about that. Rather than improve your coordination, you are more likely to develop further habits of unnecessary tension and end up with pains and aches that you never had before. The easiest way to understand the four directions is to take lessons. When you do that, you will find this chapter invaluable as an aid to understanding your lessons. While lessons cost money, they do save you time – and isn't your time worth something?

Anyway, that is how I recommend you utilize this information. You've been warned.

Definitions

Before we go on, let's be sure we agree what is meant by the 'head' and 'neck' and all the other common terms we use to describe our body parts. When we use words, we unconsciously operate on the presumption that everyone understands the same thing from the same word. I don't need to explain the fallacy of that. Just ask someone the meaning of the word 'God' and you'll get a taste of what I mean. Simple words like 'head' and 'neck', like 'God', also have different meanings to people. Alexander said:

> 'Be careful of the printed matter: you may not read it as it is written down.'

Your neck

Your neck centres around the first seven 'cervical' vertebrae shown in Figure 7.1, together with all their muscle attachments, which aren't shown. As a research project for these experiments, take time to study the extensive muscle attachments of these seven vertebrae. Some of these muscles reach right down to your lower back. On the front, they extend over the top of your rig cage as shown in Figure 7.1. The seven individual vertebrae that form the cervical spine within your neck are much wider than you think. If you push under your earlobes you will feel a hard and tender bump – that bump is actually the bony edge of your top vertebra (the atlas). The other vertebrae are not as wide, but they are still wider than most people imagine.

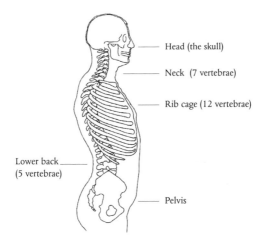

Figure 7.1 The words neck, rib cage, lower back
and pelvis can be defined in association with the
different vertebra of the spine as shown above.

Your rib cage

The next part of your body consists of the 12 'thoracic'
vertebrae which are defined through their attachment to
each of the ribs as you can see in Figure 7.1. It's not really
a cage, unless you know of a cage in which all the 'bars' can
move themselves individually? Each rib moves in a slightly
different way to the one above or below it. It isn't necessary
to know how all these movements work, only to realize how
flexible it is. Forget about iron bars; think plastic. Bone is
pliable and your ribs can move individually.

Your lower back

Your lower back consists of the last five 'lumbar' vertebrae
(also see Figure 7.2) which are differentiated partly because
none of them have a rib attached. Following them, but

hidden by the pelvis in Figure 7.1, are the fused vertebrae of the sacrum and coccyx which are wedged into the pelvis. The thing about the spine as a whole, and particularly the lower spine, is that it's enormous. Much bigger than you think. Wrap your hands around one of your upper thighs: unless you're very overweight, that, together with its muscle attachments, is about how thick your lower spine is. We've got another leg in the middle of our torso!

Your pelvis

Your pelvis consists of three bones fused together. It manipulates the weight transference of your spine through to your legs, while also serving as the foundation for muscle attachments from both legs and your lower back. An important muscle that connects this way is the psoas muscle, shown in Figure 7.2. Study this muscle: you can learn a lot about the connection between your lower back and legs by sensing this muscle's action.

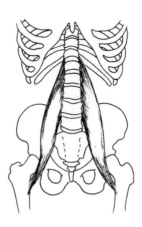

Figure 7.2 This shows the important psoas muscle that connects our legs into our lower back. Only one part of this muscle is shown.

Your torso and spine

Your torso is a collective name for your neck, rib cage, lower back and pelvis; it also includes all the guts, flesh and skin that make the shape of your body. What is your spine? It consists of all the vertebrae connected with your neck (7 vertebrae), rib cage (12 vertebrae), lower back (5 vertebrae) and the vertebrae that fuse together to form your sacral and coccyx bones.

Imagine a picture of your spine, showing its position and thickness in your torso. A lot of people think of the spine as being those bumps you can feel on your back. So they imagine the spine as being a thin little tube lying quite close to the back. Wrong! The spine is a thick supporting and integrating structure and it couldn't perform its job if it was really built as people imagine. Those bumps are the outer edges of your vertebrae, called the spinous processes, as shown on Figure 7.3. The main weight-bearing part of the spine is the 'body' of each vertebra, and that lies further in, towards the centre of your torso.

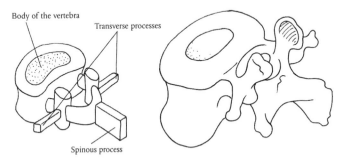

Figure 7.3 This is a typical vertebra of the spine in schematic form (left) and an example (right) of a lumbar vertebra. Note the three 'beams' called the transverse and spinous processes, on to which muscles attach.

The primary movement

All four directions concern what Alexander described as the 'true and primary movement' of your body. Put simply, the head leads and the body follows. In everything. Alexander called it the 'primary control'.

Where does your head lead your body? That's simple too. Look at Figure 7.4: either it encourages you to lengthen your body (in which case you feel free and light) or it encourages you to compress your body (in which case you feel tension and discomfort).

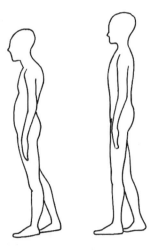

Figure 7.4 The figure on the left is shortening or compressing their body to walk, whereas the figure on the right is lengthening.

The relation of your head/neck to your body is always influencing your coordination – sometimes beneficially, but more often than not harmfully. If you get neck tension, a sore back, sore knees, breathing difficulties, repetitive strain injuries or unnecessary tension of any kind, I would bet my house that you are pulling your head back and down into your body.

Here's a little activity to experience the operation of this 'primary control' in yourself. Get down on all fours and have a friend gently take your head within their hands as shown in Figure 7.5.

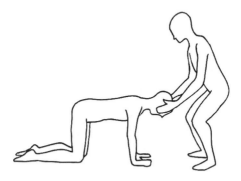

Figure 7.5 This simple activity can generate for the person crawling a clear experience of Alexander's 'primary control' principle in operation.

Now let your friend to guide you by delicately turning your head to look left or right. You will experience that you are impelled to crawl in the direction that your head is being led. Try not to go that way. Leave your head free to be led by your partner, but at the same time attempt to crawl in the opposite direction. It's near impossible, unless you can turn your head that way too. The head leads and the body follows.

PART 1: DISCOVERING THE DIRECTIONS
The preliminary stance

First, as Alexander did, get yourself at least two mirrors, as shown in Figure 7.6, so you can easily see your profile without having to twist your neck.

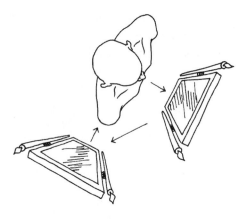

Figure 7.6 Set up two mirrors in this way so you can
observe your profile without twisting your neck.

All these experiments are done while standing, so I need to
explain your preliminary stance or posture. At the moment,
no doubt, you have many ideas about a correct and incorrect
posture. You might even try to put these into effect by
standing up straight or holding yourself more erect.

Why would anyone want to stand up straight? Because
they're slouching, of course. So the action of standing up
straight needs the slouch to come into existence, doesn't it?
Without the slouch, what need is there to stand up straight?
This means that slouching and standing up straight are
not separate; they are two sides of the same coin. For the
front of a coin to exist, the back of a coin must also come
into existence. Can you imagine a coin that doesn't have
two sides? It is no different when talking of slouching and
standing up straight. They always exist together; they are
two sides of the same thing.

As the crux of these experiments is learning to rid
yourself of the slouch altogether, this approach of standing
up straight won't work. So don't bother trying to correct
your posture in any way. Just let yourself be as you find

yourself. You may not like how you feel or look, but it's the truth. Accept it.

For these experiments, just assume your normal everyday posture.

The first direction

Having established the nature of this primary movement, the next question must be: how can my head lead me to lengthen, rather than shorten, as shown in Figure 7.4? Alexander's answer was his first direction. The words go like this: *Allow my neck to be free in such a way that my head can go forwards and up.*

My teacher Marjorie Barstow translated this whole first direction into 'Delicately move my whole head forwards and up', the 'delicately' replacing 'allow my neck to be free'. She got into a lot of trouble with more traditionally minded teachers for saying it this way. They thought putting it like this would encourage people to do the 'forwards and up' direction by tensing their necks, which is quite wrong. Marj had her reasons, and I agreed with her, but this point shows that Alexander teachers fuss a lot about words and rightly so. How you think is how you move. *Alexander work is more about your thoughts than it is about your movements.*

There is an enormous amount of information in the short sentence above. Let's start with the first six words: *Allow my neck to be free...*

This isn't a movement, it is a reminder of an important aspect of your thinking – its quality. 'Pushy' thinking induces contraction; 'delicate' thinking induces lengthening. Don't think of your mind or thoughts as somehow separate from your body's movements; your thoughts *are* how muscles behave.

All a muscle can do is contract. A muscle can't 'do' lengthening. Lengthening results when a muscle stops contracting. So *letting your neck be free* isn't something you can do, for it is the result of you *not doing* something. See Figure 3.4 again.

Sometimes Alexander work can drive you crazy – it's so contradictory to anything you've ever done with your coordination before. But have patience and keep remembering this point: you cannot 'do' any of the directions; every one of them is about *preventing* or *stopping* you from doing what you are doing. Reread Chapter 3 if you still don't get this point – it's critical to everything.

Now the next five words: ... *in such a way that...*

Some people think a free neck means you let head flop around like a rag doll. Alexander teachers don't think that. To them, a 'free neck' is one that allows your head to 'go forwards and up'; it is dynamic, alert and poised. So you free your neck *in such a way that* this result is achieved.

A 'free neck' doesn't mean 'without tension'. There has to be tension, or your head would nod off as it does when you're sleepy, because of the way it balances on your spine as shown in Figure 7.7.

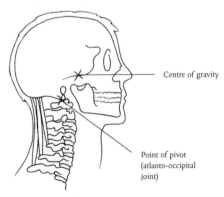

Centre of gravity

Point of pivot
(atlanto-occipital
joint)

Figure 7.7 The centre of weight of the head, called 'centre of gravity', is situated in front of the joint between the head and spine, called 'point of pivot'. For this reason, the head is naturally falling forwards all the time.

The real question is: how much tension? And the answer is: enough so that your head isn't pulled back and down, which means, by inference, that it must be going forwards and up.

Now the last seven words of the first direction: ...*my head can go forwards and up*...

Alexander didn't discover 'forwards and up'; he discovered its opposite – backwards and down. So, tempting as it might be to describe 'forwards and up', I won't do it first because it's the wrong place to start. The place for you to start is, like Alexander, to discover what its opposite 'backwards and down' actually means.

Defining movements of the head and neck

To clarify our discussion of these 'backwards and down' movements of the head and neck, I will define the terms that will be employed henceforth.

First, do this little activity: tilt only your head forward. Do it now. Did you also bend your neck forward? In 99 per cent of cases the answer is 'yes' – despite the fact that I emphasized *only* the head. What does this prove? That most people think of their neck and head as one unit – not as separate elements that combine to make movements. Actually, the top joint of the spine is at the level of your earlobes as shown in Figure 7.8 (also refer to Figure 7.7).

Now just tilt your head forwards, watching that the only movement is at that head/neck joint, called the *atlanto-occipital* joint (see Figure 7.7). You'll discover that the movement is tiny, almost negligible. If it feels big to you, look in a mirror and check whether you're bending your neck forwards as well.

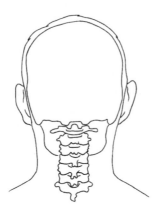

Figure 7.8 Note that our spine reaches high up
behind our jaw, reaching the level of our earlobes.

Refer to Figures 7.9, 7.10 and 7.11, which show the
critical ways you can move your head and neck. I will use
the expressions: 'head forward' (Fig 7.9a); 'head back' (Fig
7.9b); 'head tucked in' (Fig 7.11c); 'neck up' (Fig 7.10c);
'neck down' (Fig 7.10b). Spend some time to grasp the
visual meaning of these terms by comparing the illustrations
with your own head/neck relationship in the mirror in the
following two experiments until they are quite clear to you.
For simplicity, I haven't discussed rotational movements but
they will be occurring too.

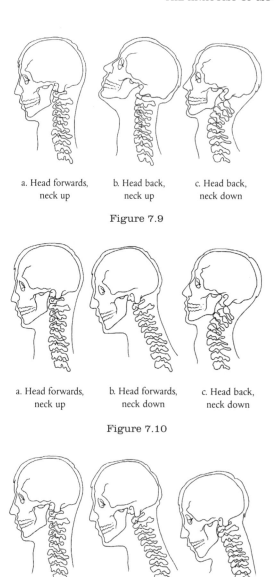

a. Head forwards,   b. Head back,   c. Head back,
   neck up   neck up   neck down

Figure 7.9

a. Head forwards,   b. Head forwards,   c. Head back,
   neck up   neck down   neck down

Figure 7.10

a. Head forwards,   b. Head forwards,   c. Head tucked in,
   neck up   neck down   neck down

Figure 7.11

First experiment: Discovering 'backwards and down'

Reread the section above, 'The preliminary stance', and assume it before beginning this experiment.

First, just look. Is your head moving? At first you might say, 'No, it's not.' You're wrong. It is moving. Look again more carefully. Be patient and keep watching until, eventually, you can see that 'Yes, my head is moving a little.' Now you are ready to begin observing your movements.

Say something and watch where your head moves. Do this experiment again, and again and again – at least 20 or 30 times – until you are sure you can see yourself doing almost the same thing every time you speak. There will be other things you are doing that are slightly different every time, but there will be one thing that is constant. Can you figure out what? No? Now you're understanding what Alexander went through. At this point he didn't see much of anything either!

What Alexander did next was a little like this. Continue watching, but now shout 'Hello!' Do this many times. Now what does your head and neck do? A lot more, I'll bet. For the final part of this experiment, start comparing the two – speaking and shouting – again many times – asking yourself if they are different. They will be, but how are they different? How do you move your head and neck each time? You need to spend several sessions on this. Remember Alexander's quote about needing discipline?

Persevere with these experiments patiently, in both activities of speaking and shouting, until you figure out what you are doing with your head and neck. Most of you doing this experiment will observe that you pull your *head back*, lifting the chin up as exclusively shown in Figure 7.9b while also dropping *your neck down* as exclusively shown in Figure 7.10b, to create a combined effect of head back and neck down as shown integrated together in Figure 7.9c. You may be one of the rarer few with your head *tucked in* while you pull your neck down as shown integrated together in Figure 7.11c.

Some readers may be wondering when they get to try moving their head forwards and up. Well, not yet. First, like Alexander, you've got to get the problem. And that means taking ample time for watching and learning about how you are coordinating yourself at the moment. Work until you are crystal clear about the movements of your head and neck. Before applying any antidotes in the form of Alexander directions, it is now important to analyze the flow-on effect that these movements have on the remainder of your coordination.

The second direction

Here's the second direction, added on to the first: *(1) Allow my neck to be free in such a way that my head can go forwards and up (2) in such a way that my body can lengthen…*

Understanding these directions is like juggling four balls at once. Now you are watching one ball and I am about to ask you to watch a second. It gets more complicated.

…*in such a way that my body can lengthen…* You don't want to think about your 'neck' in isolation as I have suggested up to this point. What your neck does is connected with the movement of your whole torso: when standing, to compensate the bending of your neck down, you will arch your torso back from the lower back, which in turn increases the inward curve at your lower back and results in thrusting your hips forward as shown in Figure 7.12b.

Second experiment: Discovering 'shortening'

Resume a 'preliminary stance' again, with your mirror set up as shown in Figure 7.6. As in the first experiment, just start by looking. The temptation is to start 'correcting' things by readjusting your stance. Resist doing that. Be still and watch. As you watch, you will notice that you can't be completely still; it's impossible. Very subtly, you are rocking back and forth and around in a circle on your two feet.

Watch that carefully for a long time, seeing if you can discern any pattern to that movement? Is it connected with your breathing at all? It may be or it may not be – that's for you to figure out. Remember, you are experimenting, so you are not supposed to be expecting anything. I will tell you some things you could see, but it is up to you to test this information for yourself. Be careful not to find what you are looking for. Find what is actually happening and see if it matches up with my description.

Now that you notice this gentle rocking movement, analyze it more carefully. For example, does the movement occur mainly at the ankle joint? Can you discern if there is any movement between the rib cage and lower back? How does this movement affect the balance of your head and neck? Here are some things you can look for.

Rib cage and torso movements

Watch the movement of your whole rib cage in standing. More likely than not you will see that while your rib cage slumps down, your whole upper torso manages to arch back from the lower back. Let's look at these two motions carefully.

First, check if your head is going back and your neck going down as in Figure 7.9c. If so, can you feel that the downward compression of your rib cage results from this pressure that your *neck down* places on it, as shown in Figure 7.12a? The rib cage slumps down under the force of the neck above it – just as happens in a good old everyday slump. However, that isn't the only thing that is happening.

Second, even as the rib cage drops into your stomach, when you rock back can you notice if your torso moves backwards in space by bending backwards at the arch of the lower back? If you feel pressure or tension in the lower back, does this tension increase at all as you rock back? Keep sensing this tension as you watch the movement of your torso and, with patience, a clear pattern will emerge.

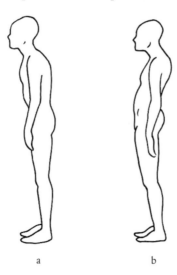

a   b

Figure 7.12 Only the collapse of the neck down with the rib cage also slumping down is shown in 7.12a, while Figure 7.12b shows how the torso bends back from the lower back, thrusting the pelvis forward and locking back the knees.

Pelvic and leg movements

Now watch the movement of your pelvis during this rocking movement of the torso. When your torso bends back from the lower back, which direction is your pelvis pushed in? Does it arch by increasing the inward curve of the lower back? Does the whole pelvis move forwards to counteract the backwards movement of the torso? If you look carefully, you might notice that both manage to happen!

Let's observe each movement as illustrated in Figure 7.13.

First, from its starting position – shown by the dotted lines – your pelvis most probably arches backwards and up, leading to an increased curve in your lower back. This concave curve in your lower back is also a result of your rib cage – shown in its starting position by the dotted lines – and your torso as a whole bending back, with your lower back as the pivot for this movement. Together, these two actions lead to an increased inward curve in your lower back and, not incidentally, greater tension and potential for pain.

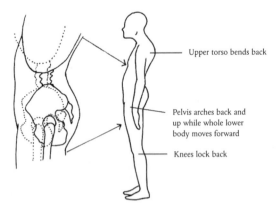

Figure 7.13 The curve in the lower back is exaggerated by the movements of the whole torso, along with the rib cage, bending back as the pelvis arches up. Both are shown in their original positions by the dotted lines.

Second, your pelvis can be moving forwards (as it arches up) by the forward movement of your legs at the ankle joint – likened to bringing your weight forward on to the front of your foot. However, your weight doesn't come forward because, to counteract this, you then lock your knees back.

Spend time analyzing what I have described (refer to Figure 7.13 to see its whole effect) by observing and sensing your own coordination. Check it out. Do you do this? Remember, we are not talking about something that is fixed; it is a continuous, subtle activity. Certainly, you can feel heavy and tight, but don't mistake that for thinking you are fixed. Tension is an activity of little movements that can be watched. Remember, it is an exquisitely subtle little dance.

By now you should have spent a good, long time observing these movements in yourself, so you are ready to experiment with the application of Alexander's antidotes in the form of the first two directions. If you haven't fully understood the previous section, please be patient, go back and continue observing your coordination until the pattern I have described above is clearer to you.

If it all seems way too subtle and complicated to you, remember my earlier advice: these experiments will be even more helpful as a support to lessons, rather than as an alternative to them. However, with a sincere and dedicated attitude, with diligence, patience, concentration and an enthusiastic attitude of open-mindedness, I also believe there is a lot you can do on your own.

Part 2: Applying the directions
Third experiment: Experiencing 'forwards'

Stand in front of the mirrors and take time to become sensitive to the gentle flow of the rocking movement described in the second experiment. Now you carefully repeat the entire analysis of the previous two experiments. To do this, Alexander worked in three steps:

1. *To analyze the conditions of use present.* First, as you rock, what does your head and neck do? Is there a *head back* movement, your chin lifting slightly up as shown in Figure 7.9c? If this happens, can you sense any increase of tension in your neck as you rock back? If so, this tells you that the muscles that can pull your *head back* are tightening. Or do you feel more that your *head tucks in* as shown in Figure 7.11c? It may feel less of a movement, more of a holding position. Spend at least five minutes sensing to your coordination – until a clear image emerges of how your head is moving at the top of your spine.

   Now, still tracking the backward movement of the head, can you feel how this causes downward pressure on your neck, pushing your neck down as shown in Figure 7.10b and 7.11c? Now, can you feel how your neck pushes down on your rib cage, causing it to slump into your body?

   While continuing to be aware of all this, track the whole movement of your torso in space. Does it sometimes fall back, causing you to bend back a little at the lower back? It will be useful here to include awareness of your breathing. Do you feel constricted? Can you discern a relationship between the movements and tension you are making with any constriction of your breath?

   Keep monitoring all this – by continually going back and checking the conditions of all these relationships – as you finally sense the action of your pelvis and legs. Is your pelvis pulling up and back increasing the arch of your lower back?

Can you sense how that goes part and parcel with the movement of your rib cage, neck and head? And as your torso bends back in space, arching at the lower back, can you feel your pelvis being thrust forwards?

Finally – as you keep an awareness of *all* of the above – watch the action of the knees. Do they brace back? When? Is it also in concert with this whole downward pattern? As you watch, can you notice that the knees lock back as your pelvis thrusts forwards?

By watching all of this activity you come to an understanding of the second step, which Alexander expressed as:

2. *To select (reason out) the means whereby a more satisfactory use could be brought about.* The 'means whereby', of course, are the Alexander directions, but they can't be exactly the same every time you employ them. Why? Because the map (your directions) isn't the territory (your coordination). What Alexander intends with this second step is for you to relate his directions to your *specific* coordination. Alexander directions are counteracting tendencies dependent upon what is perceived *as already going on.* If you don't relate them to the specifics of your coordination in any moment, you become 'Alexandroid'-like, merely imposing one set of habits upon another.

Having figured out the specifics of your coordination, now the real fun can begin. This involves applying Alexander's third and final step:

3. *To project consciously the directions required for putting these means into effect.* Start by very subtly thinking of releasing your *head forwards* (not your neck)

as you feel its backward pull. The subtle release forwards of the head only happens as you can sense the tightening of it going back. It's a question of timing. As you feel a slight increase of tension in the back of your neck – which can happen during the movement backwards and during the movement forwards – think of releasing your neck muscles in a way that allows your head to tilt forwards. As you do that, check that you aren't tightening under the chin and throat – this will happen if you tighten muscles to pull your head forwards, rather than lengthening the muscles that pulled it back.

Continue with this releasing *head forwards* by letting the muscles of the neck be free; each time there will be a little more to release. Paradoxically, the more you release the *head forwards*, the more easily you can feel it tightening back. It will never be quite the same twice in a row; that is why it is so essential to release your head forwards *in relation* to the feeling of it going back. It's why I guided you to initially spend so long doing little else but becoming familiar with your pattern of coordination. It's also why Alexander's work is so different from any other 'posture improvement' technique: you are not learning anything new; you are un-learning what you already do.

Alexander said:

> 'As soon as people come with the ideas of unlearning instead of learning, you have them in the frame of mind you want.'

Even this little experiment, if done with delicacy and precision, will manifest in a subtle improvement in the pattern of movement throughout your whole body. You may feel your breathing become less constricted, the pressure on your lower back lessening, the whole effort of standing becoming less. If you don't feel that, go back and watch more carefully and keep repeating this experiment until you can sense that this tiny release of your *head forwards* affects the whole pattern of movement. Persistence will pay off; impatience will not.

Reviewing 'forwards and up'

For these experiments you need to develop a clear definition of 'forwards and up' and how this relates to your own head/neck movements. 'Forwards' refers to the movement of your head and only your head; it does not mean you want your neck to go down. If you make that movement – that is, letting your neck go down as shown in Figure 7.11c – it looks as if you are bowing as they do in Japan. In actual fact, all *head forwards* means is preventing your head from going back as shown in Figure 7.9b. 'Head level' might be another way of putting it. We could say that if your head isn't going back, there's no reason to think of it going forwards *because it will already be doing that.*

The 'up' refers to your neck and whole body. While there's more than a hundred muscles that can pull your *neck down* as shown in Figure 7.10b, it is only by releasing those muscles that you can achieve *neck up* as shown in Figure 7.10a. It is useful to acknowledge the presence of the scalene and sterno-mastoid muscles as shown in Figure 7.14 and their role in lengthening in order that your neck can release 'up' before proceeding to the next experiment.

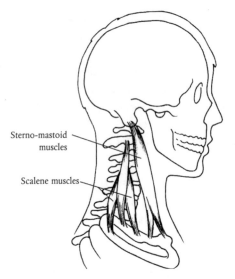

Sterno-mastoid
muscles

Scalene muscles

Figure 7.14 The combined action of the scalene
and sterno-mastoid muscles can pull your
neck down or release it up again.

Fourth experiment: Experiencing 'forwards and up'

As you are aware of tilting your *head forwards*, become aware of the forward, downward pressure that results in the *neck down* movement shown in Figure 7.11b. Can you relieve that pressure by decreasing the tension in your neck by taking your *neck up* as shown in Figure 7.9a? This can take a devil of a time to figure out. It's easy to make the neck look as if it goes 'up' (and back) if you *increase* tension – anyone can do that. But the point here is to experiment until you are able to think it up in a way that *reduces* the feeling of strain. The key is to ensure that your head continues in its *head forwards* orientation as you experiment releasing your *neck up* and back. My teacher Marj once remarked: 'You have to be very honest to do this work.'

This experiment epitomizes the reason for her remark. In your eagerness to succeed, it will be easy to delude yourself that there isn't an increase of tension in your neck. This requirement of increased ease and freedom in your neck is the guiding principle of your experiment: *you must be able to achieve even a little of this before carrying on any further.* That could take you months to figure out. Alternatively, it could happen instantly. Everyone is different – even from one pupil to the next, I am never sure how easily or not this will happen.

To succeed you need to work creatively. Here are a few tips which could help.

First, familiarize yourself thoroughly with the muscular organization of this part of your body. There is a major 'group' of muscles that run between the neck and upper chest – some are shown in Figure 7.14. It is these muscles that need to lengthen. Second, remember that while lengthening a muscle means doing less, it does not mean completely relaxing it. Third, you delicately lengthen not only so your neck is being released up from your rib cage, but additionally so your rib cage is being released away from your neck. Together, these directions result in an opening of space between your chest and neck.

If you find that you are starting to fall backwards as you apply these directions, you are ready to move on.

Fifth experiment: Experiencing 'forwards and up and lengthening'

If you are a member of the 'classic downward pull' club (see Figure 7.12b), then the reason you fall backwards is because your torso is bending back. It did that to counteract the falling forwards of your neck, but since your neck is not doing that any more, your torso is out of line. So you start to fall backwards instead.

This is a useful occurrence because, *if it doesn't happen*, either you don't need to think about this next direction (unlikely) or you're getting ahead of yourself and need to go back and play more with the direction detailed in the fourth experiment.

So now, as you counteract the tightening of your head and neck by allowing them to release *head forwards* and *neck up* (the two elements of the first direction), you add the second direction of allowing your whole torso to move forwards through space as shown by Figure 7.4b.

Using the two mirrors becomes indispensable at this point (see Figure 7.6). When you succeed in giving both these directions together – and success means reduced tension, easier breathing, a sense of tallness, lightness and ease – you will feel as though you are leaning forwards or that your bottom is sticking out at the back.

The release of your torso forwards – while still directing your *head forwards* and *neck up* – does result in arresting the movement forward of your pelvis, thus bringing your bottom back in space a little. This adds to the impression that your bottom is sticking out at the back and that you are leaning forward. To a certain extent you are right: you will be further forwards in stance from how you habitually align yourself, and your hips will not be as forward as usual, but if you look carefully in the mirror, you should see that actually you have straightened up: you're not leaning forward at all.

If you are leaning forward, then you've gone wrong somewhere. Go back over the original experiments and find the moment where you did this. Alexander had to retrace his steps this way countless times.

Alexander's Catch-22

Giving these two directions means that you are now juggling many balls, but which ball is the *first* ball when you're juggling a whole swag of them? Alexander answered that with the expression 'All together, one after the other.' It's the Catch-22 of giving directions which I've kindly saved you from until now. It goes like this: the only way to allow the rib cage to ease forwards is by directing your head forwards while lengthening up, *but* the way for your head to go forwards is by lengthening up which is caused by easing your torso forwards. It is easy to activate the second direction while you are also activating the first, but it is difficult to realize either direction unless you activate both together.

Until this point, whatever you thought was forwards and up probably wasn't forwards and up at all. In fact, forwards and up is *never* going to feel the same twice in a row if you're doing these experiments correctly. My teacher Marj always used to remind us: 'It's never going to feel the same twice. If you memorize your feelings, you'll never change.'

All the directions work like this; each one points itself towards the next one so that the sum is greater than the parts. They integrate when they occur together, one after the other. You do the first direction to cause the second direction, then you immediately project the first and the second directions in order to cause the third and so on. Alexander adopted the expression 'thinking in activity' to describe this process. He claimed that 'anyone who carries it out faithfully while trying to gain an end will find he is acquiring a new experience in what he calls "thinking"'.

Alexander spent many, many years coming to understand how all the directions work together, but you can experience this in the space of a few minutes under the skilful guidance of a teacher's hands. In these experiments, if you fail to link the directions together, it won't work. The good news is that by combining directions you can generate powerful experiences of release. The small releases you had to begin with are going to increase in their magnitude until it all begins to feel quite magnificent and magical.

What next?

One whole area I have neglected to discuss is the relationship of your arms and shoulders – which are actually the same thing – to your coordination. You will find some information in Chapter 6 under the heading 'Your left and right shoulder-arms'.

Shoulder-arms are critical in achieving what Alexander called 'widening', but, quite honestly, I would need to write a whole book to address this subject meaningfully. The more elements we combine, the greater the complexity – soon words are inadequate. How do I explain, for example, that the greatest difficulty people have is their belief that to release their shoulders they must let them drop down, when that is the very cause of why they are tight in the first place?

To release, most shoulders need to go up, not down – but not 'up' in any way that it might be conventionally conceived. Certainly not 'pulling them back' or 'lifting them up' with any tension; in a sense they release from their lower end and glide or float up. Yet that release can only be understood in a context of the various habits of misuse in our head/neck/torso. Combine what we find there with what we find our shoulders and arms doing and an almost countless variety of outcomes could result. People are unique and at some point words just can't cover all the bases.

There are four directions and I have only attempted to analyze the first two. All four directions run like this: *(1) Allow my neck to be free in such a way that my head can go forwards and up (2) in such a way that my body can lengthen (3) and widen (4) in such a way that my knees go forwards and away.*

After that, there are potentially hundreds of secondary directions you can get into. Like any great art form, there's no end to the skill you can develop.

This is an introductory book and what I have written, combined with lessons, is more than enough to keep you busy for years. Those readers who manage to work through this programme will develop an ability to generate fresh insights and will not be stopped from continuing by the lack of information on the last two directions. Alexander work is a journey, an exploration into a whole new field of enquiry, and the more you investigate, the more the results encourage you to continue. As Alexander once so aptly put it:

> 'There is so much to be seen when one reaches the point of being able to see, and the experience makes the meat it feeds upon.'

RESOURCES

Information

www.alexandertechnique.com

This site is a great resource for finding teachers, information about teacher training, articles, links to recordings and videos. It is the place to start.

Books

There are many wonderful books written about Alexander Technique, but if you are a serious reader, the first thing to do is read Alexander's own works. There are four books, in this order of publication:

Man's Supreme Inheritance.

Conscious Constructive Control of the Individual.

Use of the Self.

The Universal Constant in Living.

There are several editions and sometimes downloads available on the web, but the most authoritative and noteworthy editions, and highly recommended by me, come from Mouritz (www.mouritz.co.uk).

Here's a list of classic works published over the years, all excellent reads:

Freedom to Change: The Development and Science of the Alexander Technique by Frank Pierce Jones

The Alexander Technique: How to Use Your Body Without Stress by Dr Wilfred Barlow M.D.

Body Learning by Michael J. Gelb

How to Learn the Alexander Technique: A Manual for Students by Barbara and William Conable

The Art of Swimming by Steven Shaw and Armand d'Angour

Master the Art of Running by Malcolm Balk and Andrew Shields

EyeBody by Peter Grunwald

Golfsense by Ray Palmer

Mind and Body Stress Relief with the Alexander Technique by Richard Brennan

What Every Musician Needs to Know About the Body by Barbara Conable

This is by no means an exhaustive list, and the omission of a book does not imply it is unworthy! I suggest you select a topic you are interested in and start with that. I've also included some specialist books in the list above.

Teachers

www.ati-net.com

For Marjorie Barstow lineage teachers, a great majority can be found as members of Alexander Technique International, including my own Japanese teachers. Also articles and information on Alexander Technique.

www.stat.org.uk

The mother of all Alexander societies – here you will find teachers from all the other lineages I discuss in this book. Expect to stand in and out of chairs, and get 'tablework' from a majority of these teachers, although many will do activity work with you these days. Why not ask?

www.alexandertechnique.com

I know, I already listed it. This site, unlike me, has no axe to grind. Everyone gets to participate, so I recommend starting there to learn more. How fair's that?

The Future

www.bodychance.com

My life purpose is to create an international franchise of BodyChance Alexander Technique teachers who have a deep and comprehensive training, who follow the pedagogical approach of Marjorie Barstow and can be relied upon to deliver an experience that matches my unrelenting belief that Alexander has delivered one of the most profound scientific discoveries, ever.

Warning: Although BodyChance already runs the largest teacher education college in the world, it is in Japan! The website is Japanese. Plans are afoot to open a studio in an English-speaking country, so keep coming back. If you join BodyChance's mailing list, all my translated messages come with English at the end.

ABOUT THE AUTHOR

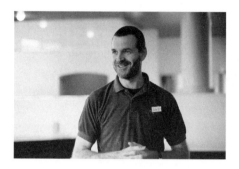

Jeremy Chance started his training as a teacher in London in 1976. Since that time, he has established himself as an internationally known and respected teacher of Alexander Technique. He has published many papers on the work, has been a featured teacher at several International Congresses of the Alexander Technique and has made innumerable appearances as a speaker in Australia, New Zealand and throughout Europe, USA and Japan.

The first milestone of his career was in 1983, when he was instrumental in establishing an Alexander Technique school for teachers in Sydney, followed by another school in Melbourne in 1987. He then founded and convened the first Australian Society of Teachers – AUSTAT – thus laying the groundwork for the profession in Alexander's country of birth.

From 1985 to 2001, Jeremy founded, published and edited *direction*, an international journal on the Alexander Technique which is still in publication. In 1999 he married and went to live permanently in Japan to raise two daughters.

In 2005 he founded his company BodyChance, which now runs the largest Alexander Technique teacher education college in the world, with studios in Tokyo and Osaka. Jeremy has personally overseen a new generation of teachers in Japan, while BodyChance continues to flourish and grow in a way the Alexander world has never seen before.

Jeremy currently divides his time between Australia, where his two daughters live, and Japan, where BodyChance operates.